Nursing Leadership and Management
REVIEW MODULE EDITION 7.0

P9-CDL-762

Contributors

Norma Jean E. Henry, MSN/Ed, RN

Mendy McMichael, DNP, MSN

Janean Johnson, MSN, RN, CNE

Agnes DiStasi, DNP, RN, CNE

Brenda S. Ball, MEd, BSN, RN

Honey C. Holman, MSN, RN

Consultants

Catherine Belden, DHSc, MSN, RN

Jenni L. Hoffman, DNP, FNP-C, CLNC

Director of content review: Kristen Lawler

Director of development: Derek Prater

Project management: Janet Hines, Nicole Burke

Coordination of content review: Norma Jean E. Henry, Mendy McMichael

Copy editing: Kelly Von Lunen, Derek Prater

Layout: Spring Lenox, Randi Hardy

Illustrations: Randi Hardy

Online media: Morgan Smith, Ron Hanson, Nicole Lobdell, Brant Stacy

Cover design: Jason Buck

Interior book design: Spring Lenox

IMPORTANT NOTICE TO THE READER

User's Guide

Welcome to the Assessment Technologies Institute® Nursing Leadership and Management Review Module Edition 7.0. The mission of ATI's Content Mastery Series® Review Modules is to provide user-friendly compendiums of nursing knowledge that will:

- Help you locate important information quickly.
- Assist in your learning efforts.
- Provide exercises for applying your nursing knowledge.
- Facilitate your entry into the nursing profession as a newly licensed nurse.

This newest edition of the Review Modules has been redesigned to optimize your learning experience. We've fit more content into less space and have done so in a way that will make it even easier for you to find and understand the information you need.

ORGANIZATION

Chapters in this Review Module use a nursing concepts organizing framework, beginning with an overview describing the central concept and its relevance to nursing. Subordinate themes are covered in outline form to demonstrate relationships and present the information in a clear, succinct manner. Some chapters have sections that group related concepts and contain their own overviews. These sections are included in the table of contents.

ACTIVE LEARNING SCENARIOS AND APPLICATION EXERCISES

Each chapter includes opportunities for you to test your knowledge and to practice applying that knowledge. Active Learning Scenario exercises pose a nursing scenario and then direct you to use an ATI Active Learning Template (included at the back of this book) to record the important knowledge a nurse should apply to the scenario. An example is then provided to which you can compare your completed Active Learning Template. The Application Exercises include NCLEX-style questions, such as multiple-choice and multiple-select items, providing you with opportunities to practice answering the kinds of questions you might expect to see on ATI assessments or the NCLEX. After the Application Exercises, an answer key is provided, along with rationales.

NCLEX® CONNECTIONS

To prepare for the NCLEX, it is important to understand how the content in this Review Module is connected to the NCLEX test plan. You can find information on the detailed test plan at the National Council of State Boards of Nursing's website, www.ncsbn.org. When reviewing content in this Review Module, regularly ask yourself, "How does this content fit into the test plan, and what types of questions related to this content should I expect?"

To help you in this process, we've included NCLEX Connections at the beginning of each unit and with each question in the Application Exercises Answer Keys. The NCLEX Connections at the beginning of each unit point out areas of the detailed test plan that relate to the content within that unit. The NCLEX Connections attached to the Application Exercises Answer Keys demonstrate how each exercise fits within the detailed content outline. These NCLEX Connections will help you understand how the detailed content outline is organized, starting with major client needs categories and subcategories and followed by related content areas and tasks. The major client needs categories are:

- Safe and Effective Care Environment
  - Management of Care
  - Safety and Infection Control
- Health Promotion and Maintenance
- Psychosocial Integrity
- Physiological Integrity
  - Basic Care and Comfort
  - Pharmacological and Parenteral Therapies
  - Reduction of Risk Potential
  - Physiological Adaptation

An NCLEX Connection might, for example, alert you that content within a chapter is related to:

- Management of Care
  - Advance Directives
    - Provide clients with information about advance directives.

QSEN COMPETENCIES

As you use the Review Modules, you will note the integration of the Quality and Safety Education for Nurses (QSEN) competencies throughout the chapters. These competencies are integral components of the curriculum of many nursing programs in the United States and prepare you to provide safe, high-quality care as a newly licensed nurse. Icons appear to draw your attention to the six QSEN competencies.

Safety: The minimization of risk factors that could cause injury or harm while promoting quality care and maintaining a secure environment for clients, self, and others.

Patient-Centered Care: The provision of caring and compassionate, culturally sensitive care that addresses clients' physiological, psychological, sociological, spiritual, and cultural needs, preferences, and values.

Evidence-Based Practice: The use of current knowledge from research and other credible sources, on which to base clinical judgment and client care.

Informatics: The use of information technology as a communication and information-gathering tool that supports clinical decision-making and scientifically based nursing practice.

Quality Improvement: Care related and organizational processes that involve the development and implementation of a plan to improve health care services and better meet clients' needs.

Teamwork and Collaboration: The delivery of client care in partnership with multidisciplinary members of the health care team to achieve continuity of care and positive client outcomes.

ICONS

Icons are used throughout the Review Module to draw your attention to particular areas. Keep an eye out for these icons.

Ⓝ This icon is used for NCLEX Connections.

Ⓖ This icon indicates gerontological considerations, or knowledge specific to the care of older adult clients.

Q𝐬 This icon is used for content related to safety and is a QSEN competency. When you see this icon, take note of safety concerns or steps that nurses can take to ensure client safety and a safe environment.

Q𝐏𝐂𝐂 This icon is a QSEN competency that indicates the importance of a holistic approach to providing care.

Q𝐄𝐁𝐏 This icon, a QSEN competency, points out the integration of research into clinical practice.

Q𝐈 This icon is a QSEN competency and highlights the use of information technology to support nursing practice.

Q𝐐𝐈 This icon is used to focus on the QSEN competency of integrating planning processes to meet clients' needs.

Q𝐓𝐂 This icon highlights the QSEN competency of care delivery using an interprofessional approach.

M◊ This icon appears at the top-right of pages and indicates availability of an online media supplement, such as a graphic, animation, or video. If you have an electronic copy of the Review Module, this icon will appear alongside clickable links to media supplements. If you have a hard copy version of the Review Module, visit www.atitesting.com for details on how to access these features.

FEEDBACK

ATI welcomes feedback regarding this Review Module. Please provide comments to comments@atitesting.com.

Table of Contents

When reviewing the following chapter, keep in mind the relevant topics and tasks of the NCLEX outline, in particular:

Client Needs: Management of Care

ASSIGNMENT, DELEGATION AND SUPERVISION
Evaluate delegated tasks to ensure correct completion of activity.

Evaluate effectiveness of staff members' time management skills.

CASE MANAGEMENT: Provide cost effective care.

CONCEPTS OF MANAGEMENT: Manage conflict among clients and health care staff.

ESTABLISHING PRIORITIES: Apply knowledge of pathophysiology when establishing priorities for interventions with multiple clients.

PERFORMANCE IMPROVEMENT (QUALITY IMPROVEMENT): Participate in performance improvement/quality improvement processes.

Managing Client Care

Managing client care requires leadership and management skills and knowledge to effectively coordinate and carry out client care.

To effectively manage client care, a nurse must develop knowledge and skills in several areas, including leadership, management, critical thinking, clinical reasoning, clinical judgment, prioritization, time management, assigning, delegating, supervising, staff education, quality improvement, performance appraisal, peer review, disciplinary action, conflict resolution, and cost-effective care.

Leadership and management

- Leadership and management are concepts that are integral to effective management and motivation of staff and clients.
- Management is the process of planning, organizing, directing, and coordinating the work within an organization.
- Leadership is the ability to inspire others to achieve a desired outcome.
- Effective managers usually possess good leadership skills. However, effective leaders are not always in a management position.
- Managers have formal positions of power and authority. Leaders might have only the informal power afforded them by their peers.
- One cannot be a leader without followers.
- A number of theories describe the characteristics of a leader. Behavioral theories describe leadership styles. Transactional and transformational leadership theories contrast two types of leaders. The emotionally intelligent leader displays sensitivity when interacting with others.

LEADERSHIP

LEADERSHIP STYLES

Most can be categorized as authoritative, democratic, or laissez-faire. The nurse might need to use any of these leadership styles depending on the situation.

Authoritative

- Makes decisions for the group.
- Motivates by coercion.
- Communication occurs down the chain of command.
- Work output by staff is usually high: good for crisis situations and bureaucratic settings.
- Effective for employees with little or no formal education.

Democratic

- Includes the group when decisions are made. Q^{rc}
- Motivates by supporting staff achievements.
- Communication occurs up and down the chain of command.
- Work output by staff is usually of good quality: good when cooperation and collaboration are necessary.

Laissez-faire

- Makes very few decisions, and does little planning.
- Motivation is largely the responsibility of individual staff members.
- Communication occurs up and down the chain of command and between group members.
- Work output is low unless an informal leader evolves from the group.
- Effective with professional employees.

CHARACTERISTICS OF LEADERS

- **Initiative**
- **Inspiration**
- **Energy**
- **Positive attitude**
- **Communication skills**
- **Respect**
- **Problem-solving and critical-thinking skills**
  - Leaders have a combination of personality traits and leadership skills.
    - Great leaders were once thought to be born with skills that could not be acquired.
    - Contemporary leadership theory supports the belief that leaders can develop the necessary skills.
  - Leaders influence willing followers to move toward a goal.
  - Leaders have goals that might not reflect those of the organization.
  - **Transformational leaders** empower followers to assume responsibility for a communal vision, and personal development is a secondary outcome.
  - **Transactional leaders** focus on immediate problems, maintaining the status quo and using rewards to motivate followers.

Emotional intelligence

- Emotional intelligence is the ability of an individual to perceive and manage the emotions of self and others.
- The nurse must be able to perceive and understand his own emotions and the emotions of the client and family in order to provide client-centered care. Qᴘᴄᴄ
- Emotional intelligence is also an important characteristic of the successful nurse leader.
- Emotional intelligence is developed through understanding the concept and applying it to practice in everyday situations.

The emotionally intelligent leader:
- Has insight into the emotions of members of the team.
- Understands the perspective of others.
- Encourages constructive criticism and is open to new ideas.
- Is able to maintain focus while multitasking.
- Manages emotions and channels them in a positive direction, which in turn helps the team accomplish its goals.
- Is committed to the delivery of high-quality client care.
- Refrains from judgment in controversial or emotionally charged situations until facts are gathered.

MANAGEMENT

The five major management functions are planning, organizing, staffing, directing, and controlling.

PLANNING: The decisions regarding what needs to be done, how it will be done, and who is going to do it

ORGANIZING: The organizational structure that determines the lines of authority, channels of communication, and where decisions are made

STAFFING: The acquisition and management of adequate staff and staffing mix

DIRECTING: The leadership role assumed by a manager that influences and motivates staff to perform assigned roles

CONTROLLING: The evaluation of staff performance and evaluation of unit goals to ensure identified outcomes are being met

CHARACTERISTICS OF MANAGERS

- Hold formal positions of authority and power
- Possess clinical expertise
- Network with members of the team
- Coach subordinates
- Make decisions about the function of the organization, including resources, budget, hiring, and firing

Critical thinking

Critical thinking is used when analyzing client issues and problems. Thinking skills include interpretation, analysis, evaluation, inference and explanation. These skills assist the nurse to determine the most appropriate action to take.
- Critical thinking reflects upon the meaning of statements, examines available data, and uses reason to make informed decisions.
- Critical thinking is necessary to reflect and evaluate from a broader scope of view.
- Sometimes one must think "outside the box" to find solutions that are best for clients, staff, and the organization.

Clinical reasoning

- Clinical reasoning is the mental process used when analyzing the elements of a clinical situation and using analysis to make a decision. The nurse continues to use clinical reasoning to make decisions as the client's situation changes.
- Clinical reasoning supports the clinical decision-making process by:
  - Guiding the nurse through the process of assessing and compiling data.
  - Selecting and discarding data based on relevance.
  - Using nursing knowledge to make decisions about client care. Problem solving is a part of decision-making.

Clinical judgment

- Clinical judgment is the decision made regarding a course of action based on a critical analysis of data.
- Clinical judgment considers the client's needs when deciding to take an action, or modify an intervention based on the client's response.
- The nurse uses clinical judgment to:
  - Analyze data and related evidence.
  - Ascertain the meaning of the data and evidence.
  - Apply knowledge to a clinical situation.
  - Determine client outcomes desired and/or achieved as indicated by evidence-based practices. Qᴇʙᴘ

PRIORITIZATION AND TIME MANAGEMENT

- Nurses must continuously set and reset priorities in order to meet the needs of multiple clients and to maintain client safety. Qs
- Priority setting requires that decisions be made regarding the order in which:
  - Clients are seen.
  - Assessments are completed.
  - Interventions are provided.
  - Steps in a client procedure are completed.
  - Components of client care are completed.
- Establishing priorities in nursing practice requires that the nurse make these decisions based on evidence obtained:
  - During shift reports and other communications with members of the health care team.
  - Through careful review of documents.
  - By continuously and accurately collecting client data.

PRIORITIZATION PRINCIPLES IN CLIENT CARE

Prioritize systemic before local ("life before limb").

> Prioritizing interventions for a client in shock over interventions for a client who has a localized limb injury

Prioritize acute (less opportunity for physical adaptation) before chronic (greater opportunity for physical adaptation).

> Prioritizing the care of a client who has a new injury/illness (e.g., mental confusion, chest pain) or an acute exacerbation of a previous illness over the care of a client who has a long-term chronic illness

Prioritize actual problems before potential future problems.

> Prioritizing administration of medication to a client experiencing acute pain over ambulation of a client at risk for thrombophlebitis

Listen carefully to clients and don't assume.

> Asking a client who has a new diagnosis of diabetes mellitus what he feels is most important to learn about disease management.

Recognize and respond to trends vs. transient findings.

> Recognizing a gradual deterioration in a client's level of consciousness and/or Glasgow Coma Scale score

Recognize indications of medical emergencies and complications vs. expected findings.

> Recognizing indications of increasing intracranial pressure in a client who has a new diagnosis of a stroke vs. the findings expected following a stroke

Apply clinical knowledge to procedural standards to determine the priority action.

> Recognizing that the timing of administration of antidiabetic and antimicrobial medications is more important than administration of some other medications

PRIORITY SETTING FRAMEWORKS

Maslow's hierarchy (1.1) QPCC

The nurse should consider this hierarchy of human needs when prioritizing interventions. For example, the nurse should prioritize a client's:
- Need for airway, oxygenation (or breathing), circulation, and potential for disability over need for shelter.
- Need for a safe and secure environment over a need for socialization.

Airway breathing circulation (ABC) framework

- The ABC framework identifies, in order, the three basic needs for sustaining life.
  - An open airway is necessary for breathing, so it is the highest priority.
  - Breathing is necessary for oxygenation of the blood to occur.
  - Circulation is necessary for oxygenated blood to reach the body's tissues.
- The severity of manifestations should also be considered when determining priorities. A severe circulation problem can take priority over a minor breathing problem.
- Some frameworks also include a "D" for disability and "E" for exposure

1.1 Maslow's hierarchy of needs

Self-actualization
Self-esteem
Love and belonging
Safety and security
Physiological

PRIORITY INTERVENTIONS
- **First: Airway**
  - Identify an airway concern (obstruction, stridor).
  - Establish a patent airway if indicated.
  - Recognize that 3 to 5 min without oxygen causes irreversible brain damage secondary to cerebral anoxia.
- **Second: Breathing**
  - Assess the effectiveness of breathing (apnea, depressed respiratory rate).
  - Intervene as appropriate (reposition, administer naloxone).
- **Third: Circulation**
  - Identify circulation concern (hypotension, dysrhythmia, inadequate cardiac output, compartment syndrome).
  - Institute appropriate actions to reverse or minimize circulatory alteration.
- **Fourth: Disability**
  - Assess for current or evolving disability (neurological deficits, stroke in evolution).
  - Implement actions to slow down development of disability.
- **Fifth: Exposure**
  - Remove the client's clothing to allow for a complete assessment or resuscitation
  - Implement measures to reduce the risk for hypothermia by providing warm blankets and IV solutions and using a heating device if needed.

Safety/risk reduction Qs

- Look first for a safety risk. For example, is there a finding that suggests a risk for airway obstruction, hypoxia, bleeding, infection, or injury?
- Next ask, "What's the risk to the client?" and "How significant is the risk compared to other posed risks?"
- Give priority to responding to whatever finding poses the greatest (or most imminent) risk to the client's physical well-being.

Assessment/data collection first

Use the nursing process to gather pertinent information prior to making a decision regarding a plan of action. For example, determine if additional information is needed prior to calling the provider to ask for pain medication for a client.

Survival potential

- Use this framework for situations in which health resources are extremely limited (mass casualty, disaster triage).
- Give priority to clients who have a reasonable chance of survival with prompt intervention. Clients who have a limited likelihood of survival even with intense intervention are assigned the lowest priority.

Least restrictive/least invasive

- Select interventions that maintain client safety while posing the least amount of restriction to the client. For example, if a client who has a high fall risk index is getting out of bed without assistance, move the client closer to the nurses' work area rather than choosing to apply restraints.
- Select interventions that are the least invasive. For example, bladder training for the incontinent client is a better option than an indwelling urinary catheter.

Acute vs. chronic, urgent vs. nonurgent, stable vs. unstable

- A client who has an acute problem takes priority over a client who has a chronic problem.
- A client who has an urgent need takes priority over a client who has a nonurgent need.
- A client who has unstable findings takes priority over a client who has stable findings.

TIME MANAGEMENT

Organize care according to client care needs and priorities. Qᴘᴄᴄ
- What must be done immediately (administration of analgesic or antiemetic, assessment of unstable client)?
- What must be done by a specific time to ensure client safety, quality care, and compliance with facility policies and procedures (routine medication administration, vital signs, blood glucose monitoring)?
- What must be done by the end of the shift (ambulation of the client, discharge and/or discharge teaching, dressing change)?
- What can the nurse delegate?
  - What tasks can only the RN perform?
  - What client care responsibilities can the nurse delegate to other health care team members, such as practical nurses (PNs) and assistive personnel (APs)?

Use time-saving strategies and avoid time wasters. (1.2)
- **Good time management**
  - Facilitates greater productivity.
  - Decreases work-related stress.
  - Helps ensure the provision of quality and appropriately prioritized client care.
  - Enhances satisfaction with care provided.
- **Poor time management**
  - Impairs productivity.
  - Leads to feelings of being overwhelmed and stressed.
  - Increases omission of important tasks.
  - Creates dissatisfaction with care provided.

Time management is a cyclic process.

- Time initially spent developing a plan will save time later and help to avoid management by crisis.
- Set goals and plan care based on established priorities and thoughtful utilization of resources.
- Complete one client care task before beginning the next, starting with the highest priority task.
- Reprioritize remaining tasks based on continual reassessment of client care needs.
- At the end of the day, perform a time analysis and determine if time was used wisely.

TIME MANAGEMENT AND TEAMWORK

- Be cognizant of assistance needed by other health care team members.
- Offer to help when unexpected crises occur.
- Assist other team members with provision of care when experiencing a period of down time.

TIME MANAGEMENT AND SELF-CARE

- Take time for yourself.
- Schedule time for breaks and meals.
- Take physical and mental breaks from work and the unit.

Assigning, delegating, and supervising

Assigning is the process of transferring the authority, accountability, and responsibility of client care to another member of the health care team. Q℡

Delegating is the process of transferring the authority and responsibility to another team member to complete a task, while retaining the accountability.

Supervising is the process of directing, monitoring, and evaluating the performance of tasks by another member of the health care team. RNs are responsible for the supervision of client care tasks delegated to APs and PNs.

Nurses must delegate appropriately and supervise adequately to ensure that clients receive safe, quality care. **(1.3)** Qs

- Delegation decisions are based on individual client needs, facility policies and job descriptions, state nurse practice acts, and professional standards. The nurse should consider legal/ethical concerns when assigning and delegating.
- The nurse leader should recognize limitations and use available information and resources to make the best possible decisions at the time. The nurse must remember that it is his responsibility to ensure that clients receive safe, effective nursing care.
- Nurses must follow the ANA codes of standards in delegating and assigning tasks.

1.2 Time management examples

Time savers

Documenting nursing interventions as soon as possible after completion to facilitate accurate and thorough documentation

Grouping activities that are to be performed on the same client or are in close physical proximity to prevent unnecessary walking

Estimating how long each activity will take and planning accordingly

Mentally envisioning the procedure to be performed and gathering all equipment prior to entering the client's room

Taking time to plan care and taking priorities into consideration

Delegating activities to other staff when client care workload is beyond what can be handled by one nurse

Enlisting the aid of other staff when a team approach is more efficient than an individual approach

Completing more difficult or strenuous tasks when energy level is high

Avoiding interruptions and graciously but assertively saying "no" to unreasonable or poorly timed requests for help

Setting a realistic standard for completion of care and level of performance within the constraints of assignment and resources

Completing one task before beginning another task

Breaking large tasks into smaller tasks to make them more manageable

Using an organizational sheet to plan care

Using breaks to socialize with staff

Time wasters

Documenting at the end of the shift all client care provided and assessments done

Making repeated trips to the supply room for equipment

Providing care as opportunity arises regardless of other responsibilities

Missing equipment when preparing to perform a procedure

Failing to plan or managing by crisis

Being reluctant to delegate or underdelegating

Not asking for help when needed or trying to provide all client care independently

Procrastinating: delaying time-consuming, less desirable tasks until late in the shift

Agreeing to help other team members with lower priority tasks when time is already compromised

Setting unrealistic standards for completion of care and level of performance within constraints of assignment and resources

Starting several tasks at once and not completing tasks before starting others

Not addressing low level of skill competency, increasing time on task

Providing care without a written plan

Socializing with staff during client care time

ASSIGNING

Assigning is performed in a downward or lateral manner with regard to members of the health care team.

CLIENT FACTORS

- Condition of the client and level of care needed
- Specific care needs (cardiac monitoring, mechanical ventilation)
- Need for special precautions (isolation precautions, fall precautions, seizure precautions)
- Procedures requiring a significant time commitment (extensive dressing changes or wound care)

HEALTH CARE TEAM FACTORS

- Knowledge and skill level of team members
- Amount of supervision necessary
- Staffing mix (RNs, PNs, AP)
- Nurse-to-client ratio
- Experience with similar clients
- Familiarity of staff member with unit

ADDITIONAL FACTORS

When a nurse receives an unsafe assignment, she should take the following actions.
- Bring the unsafe assignment to the attention of the scheduling/charge nurse and negotiate a new assignment.
- If no resolution is arrived at, take the concern up the chain of command.
- If a satisfactory resolution is still not arrived at, the nurse should file a written protest to the assignment, such as an assignment despite objection (ADO) or document of practice situation (DOPS) with the appropriate administrator.
- Failure to accept the assignment without following the proper channels can be considered client abandonment.

1.3 The health care team

LICENSED PERSONNEL: Nurses who have completed a course of study, successfully passed either the NCLEX-PN® or NCLEX-RN® exam, and have a nursing license issued by a board of nursing.

ASSISTIVE PERSONNEL: Specifically trained to function in an assistive role to licensed nurses in client care activities.

These individuals can be nursing personnel, such as certified nursing assistants (CNAs) or certified medical assistants (CMAs), or they can be nonnursing personnel to whom nursing activities can be delegated, such as dialysis technicians, monitor technicians, and phlebotomists.

Some health care entities can differentiate between nurse and nonnurse assistive personnel by using the acronym NAP for nursing assistive personnel.

DELEGATING AND SUPERVISING

A licensed nurse is responsible for providing clear directions when a task is initially delegated and for periodic reassessment and evaluation of the outcome of the task.
- RNs may delegate to other RNs, PNs, and APs.
  - RNs must be knowledgeable about the applicable state nurse practice act and regulations regarding the use of PNs and APs.
  - RNs must delegate tasks so that they can complete higher level tasks that only RNs can perform. This allows more efficient use of all members of the health care team. Qᴛᴄ
- PNs may delegate to other PNs and APs.

DELEGATION FACTORS

- Nurses can only delegate tasks appropriate for the skill and education level of the health care team member who is receiving the assignment.
- RNs cannot delegate the nursing process, client education, or tasks that require clinical judgment to PNs or AP.

TASK FACTORS

Prior to delegating client care, consider the following.

Predictability of outcome
- Will the completion of the task have a predictable outcome?
- Is it a routine treatment?
- Is it a new treatment?

Potential for harm
- Is there a chance that something negative can happen to the client (risk for bleeding, risk for aspiration)?
- Is the client unstable?

Complexity of care
- Are complex tasks required as a part of the client's care?
- Is the delegatee legally able to perform the task and does he have the skills necessary?

Need for problem solving and innovation
- Is nursing judgment required while performing the task?
- Does it require nursing assessment skills?

Level of interaction with the client
- Is there a need to provide psychosocial support or education during the performance of the task?

1.4 Examples of tasks nurses may delegate to practical nurses and assistive personnel
(provided the facility's policy and state's practice guidelines permit)

TO PN	TO AP	
Monitoring findings (as input to the RN's ongoing assessment)	Activities of daily living (ADLs)	Positioning
Reinforcing client teaching from a standard care plan	Bathing	Routine tasks
Performing tracheostomy care	Grooming	Bed making
Suctioning	Dressing	Specimen collection
Checking NG tube patency	Toileting	Intake and output
Administering enteral feedings	Ambulating	Vital signs (for stable clients)
Inserting a urinary catheter	Feeding (without swallowing precautions)	
Administering medication (excluding IV medication in some states)		

DELEGATEE FACTORS

Considerations for selection of an appropriate delegatee include the following.
- Education, training, and experience
- Knowledge and skill to perform the task
- Level of critical thinking required to complete the task
- Ability to communicate with others as it pertains to the task
- Demonstrated competence
- The delegatee's culture
- Agency policies and procedures and licensing legislation (state nurse practice acts)

DELEGATION AND SUPERVISION GUIDELINES

- Use nursing judgment and knowledge related to the scope of practice and delegatee's skill level when delegating.
- Use the five rights of delegation (1.5)
  - What tasks the nurse delegate (right task)
  - Under what circumstances (right circumstance)
  - To whom (right person)
  - What information should be communicated (right direction/communication)
  - How to supervise/evaluate (right supervision/evaluation)

Right task

- Identify what tasks are appropriate to delegate for each specific client.
- A right task is repetitive, requires little supervision, and is relatively noninvasive for the client.
- Delegate tasks to appropriate levels of team members (PN, AP) based on standards of practice, legal and facility guidelines, and available resources.

RIGHT TASK: Delegate an AP to assist a client who has pneumonia to use a bedpan.

WRONG TASK: Delegate an AP to administer a nebulizer treatment to a client who has pneumonia.

1.5 The five rights of delegation

RIGHT task
RIGHT circumstance
RIGHT person
RIGHT direction and communication
RIGHT supervision and evaluation

Right circumstance

- Assess the health status and complexity of care required by the client.
- Match the complexity of care demands to the skill level of the health care team member.
- Consider the workload of the team member.

RIGHT CIRCUMSTANCE: Delegate an AP to measure the vital signs of a client who is postoperative and stable.

WRONG CIRCUMSTANCE: Delegate an AP to measure the vital signs of a client who is postoperative and received naloxone to reverse respiratory depression.

Right person

- Assess and verify the competency of the health care team member.
  - The task must be within the team member's scope of practice.
  - The team member must have the necessary competence/training.
- Continually review the performance of the team member and determine care competency.
- Assess team member performance based on standards and, when necessary, take steps to remediate a failure to meet standards.

RIGHT PERSON: Delegate an PN to administer enteral feedings to a client who has a head injury.

WRONG PERSON: Delegate an AP to administer enteral feedings to a client who has a head injury.

Right direction/communication

Communicate either in writing or orally.
- Data that needs to be collected
- Method and time line for reporting, including when to report concerns/findings
- Specific task(s) to be performed; client-specific instructions
- Expected results, time lines, and expectations for follow-up communication

> **RIGHT DIRECTION AND COMMUNICATION:**
> Delegate an AP to assist Mr. Martin in room 312 with a shower before 0900.

> **WRONG DIRECTION AND COMMUNICATION:**
> Delegate an AP to assist Mr. Martin in room 312 with morning hygiene.

Right supervision/evaluation Q™C

The delegating nurse must:
- Provide supervision, either directly or indirectly (assigning supervision to another licensed nurse).
- Provide clear directions and expectations of the task to be performed (time frames, what to report).
- Monitor performance.
- Provide feedback.
- Intervene if necessary (unsafe clinical practice).
- Evaluate the client and determine if client outcomes were met.
- Evaluate client care tasks and identify needs for quality improvement activities and/or additional resources.

> **RIGHT SUPERVISION:** Delegate the ambulation of a client to an AP. Observe the AP to ensure safe ambulation of the client, and provide positive feedback to the AP after completion of the task.

> **WRONG SUPERVISION:** Delegate the ambulation of a client to an AP without supervision to determine the need for intervention and failing to provide feedback to the AP.

SUPERVISION

Occurs after delegation. A supervisor oversees a staff member's performance of delegated activities and determines if:
- Completion of tasks is on schedule.
- Performance was at a satisfactory level.
- Unexpected findings were documented and reported.
- Assistance is needed to complete assigned tasks in a timely manner.
- Assignment should be re-evaluated and possibly changed.

Staff education

Staff education refers to the nurse's involvement in the orientation, socialization, education, and training of fellow health care workers to ensure the competence of all staff and to help them meet standards set forth by the facility and accrediting bodies. The process of staff education is also referred to as staff development.
- The quality of client care provided is directly related to the education and level of competency of health care providers. Q EBP
- The nurse leader has a responsibility in maintaining competent staff.
- Nurse leaders work with a unique, diverse workforce. The nurse should respect and recognize the health care team's diversity. Q™C

ORIENTATION

Orientation helps newly licensed nurses translate the knowledge, skills, and attitudes learned in nursing school into practice.

ORIENTATION TO THE INSTITUTION

- The newly licensed nurse is introduced to the philosophy, mission, and goals of the institution and department.
- Policies and procedures that are based on institutional standards are reviewed.
- Use of and access to the institution's computer system is a significant focus.
- Safety and security protocols are emphasized in relation to the nurse's role.

ORIENTATION TO THE UNIT

- Classroom orientation usually moves onto the unit and is continued with an assigned preceptor.
- Preceptors assist in orienting newly licensed nurses to a unit and supervising their performance and acquisition of skills.
- Preceptors are usually assigned to newly licensed nurses for a limited amount of time.
- Mentors can also serve as a newly licensed nurse's preceptor, but their relationship usually lasts longer and focuses more on assumption of the professional role and relationships, as well as socialization to practice.
- Coaches establish a collaborative relationship to help a nurse establish specific individual goals. The relationship is often task related and typically time limited.

SOCIALIZATION

Socialization is the process by which a person learns a new role and the values and culture of the group within which that role is implemented.

- Successful socialization helps new staff members fit in with already established staff on a client care unit.
- Staff development educators and unit managers can begin this process during interviewing and orientation.
- Nurse preceptors/mentors are frequently used to assist newly licensed nurses with this process on the clinical unit.

EDUCATION AND TRAINING

Staff education, or staff development, is the process by which a staff member gains knowledge and skills. The goal of staff education is to ensure that staff members have and maintain the most current knowledge and skills necessary to meet the needs of clients. **(1.6)**

Steps in providing educational programs

Educational programs should be provided using the following sequence. ⓆEBP

1. Identify and respond: To identify need for knowledge or skill proficiency

2. Analyze: Deficiencies, and develop learning objectives to meet need

3. Research: Resources available to address learning objectives based on evidence-based practice

4. Plan: Program to address objectives using available resources

5. Implement: Program(s) at time conducive to staff attendance; consider online learning modules

6. Evaluate: Use materials and observations to measure behavior changes secondary to learning objectives

Improved nursing ability

An increase in knowledge and competence is the goal of staff education.

Competence is the ability of an employee to meet the requirements of a particular role at an established level of performance. Nurses usually progress through several stages of proficiency as they gain experience in a particular area.

The five stages of nursing ability Patricia Benner (1984) identified five stages of nursing ability, which are based on level of competence. Level of competence is directly related to length of time in practice and exposure to clinical situations. When nurses move to a new clinical setting that requires acquisition of new skills and knowledge, their level of competence will return to a lower stage. **(1.7)**

1.6 Staff education

CHARACTERISTICS	IDENTIFIED/ PROVIDED BY
Involves methods appropriate to learning domain and learning styles of staff.	Peers, unit managers, staff development educators
Initiated in specific situations	
• New policies or procedures implemented • New equipment becomes available • Educational need identified	Unit managers, staff development educators
Can focus on one-on-one approach	Unit manager, charge nurse, preceptor
Can use "just in time" training to meet immediate needs for client care	Staff members, supervisors
Higher education degree or certification	Staff

1.7 Five stages of nursing ability

Novice nurse
Novice nurses can be students or newly licensed nurses who have minimal clinical experience. They approach situations from theoretical perspective relying on context-free facts and established guidelines. Rules govern practice.

Advanced beginner
Most new nurses function at the level of the advanced beginner. They practice independently in the performance of many tasks and can make some clinical judgments. They begin to rely on prior experience to make practice decisions.

Competent nurse
These are usually nurses who have been in practice for 2 to 3 years. They demonstrate increasing levels of skill and proficiency and clinical judgment. They exhibit the ability to organize and plan care using abstract and analytical thinking. They can anticipate the long-term outcomes of personal actions.

Proficient nurse
These are nurses who have a significant amount of experience upon which to base their practice. Enhanced observational abilities allow nurses to be able to conceptualize situations more holistically. Well-developed critical thinking and decision-making skills allow nurses to recognize and respond to unexpected changes.

Expert nurse
Expert nurses have garnered a wealth of experience so they can view situations holistically and process information efficiently. They make decisions using an advanced level of intuition and analytical ability. They do not need to rely on rules to comprehend a situation and take action.

Source: http://www.scribd.com/doc/27103958/Benner-Theory-Novice-to-Expert

Quality improvement

- Quality improvement (performance improvement, quality control) is the process used to identify and resolve performance deficiencies. Quality improvement includes measuring performance against a set of predetermined standards. In health care, these standards are set by the facility and consider accrediting and professional standards. Qᴏɪ
- Standards of care should reflect optimal goals and be based on evidence.
- The quality improvement process focuses on assessment of outcomes and determines ways to improve the delivery of quality care. All levels of employees are involved in the quality improvement process.
- The Joint Commission's accreditation standards require institutions to show evidence of quality improvement in order to attain accreditation status.

QUALITY IMPROVEMENT PROCESS

The quality improvement process begins with identification of standards and outcome indicators based on evidence.

Outcome (clinical) indicators reflect desired client outcomes related to the standard under review. Qᴇʙᴘ

Structure indicators reflect the setting in which care is provided and the available human and material resources.

Process indicators reflect how client care is provided and are established by policies and procedures (clinical practice guidelines).

Benchmarks are goals that are set to determine at what level the outcome indicators should be met.

While process indicators provide important information about how a procedure is being carried out, an outcome indicator measures whether that procedure is effective in meeting the desired benchmark. For example, the use of incentive spirometers in postoperative clients can be determined to be 92% (process indicator), but the rate of postoperative pneumonia can be determined to be 8% (outcome indicator). If the benchmark is set at 5%, the benchmark for that outcome indicator is not being met and the structure and process variables need to be analyzed to identify potential areas for improvement.

STEPS IN THE QUALITY IMPROVEMENT PROCESS

A standard is developed and approved by a facility committee.

- Standards are made available to employees by way of policies and procedures.
- Quality issues are identified by staff, management, or risk management department.
- An interprofessional team is developed to review the issue.
- The current state of structure and process related to the issue is analyzed.
- Data collection methods are determined.
  - Quantitative methods are primarily used in the data collection process, although client interview is also an option.
- Data is collected, analyzed, and compared with the established benchmark.
- If the benchmark is not met, possible influencing factors are determined. A root cause analysis can be done to critically assess all factors that influence the issue. A root cause analysis: Qᴇʙᴘ
  - Focuses on variables that surround the consequence of an action or occurrence.
  - Is commonly done for sentinel events (client death, client care resulting in serious physical injury) but can also be done as part of the quality improvement process.
  - Investigates the consequence and possible causes.
  - Analyzes the possible causes and relationships that can exist.
  - Determines additional influences at each level of relationship.
  - Determines the root cause or causes.
- Potential solutions or corrective actions are analyzed and one is selected for implementation.
- Educational or corrective action is implemented.
- The issue is reevaluated at a preestablished time to determine the efficacy of the solution or corrective action.

Audits

Audits can produce valuable quantitative data.

Types of audits

- Structure audits evaluate the influence of elements that exist separate from or outside of the client-staff interaction.
- Process audits review how care was provided and assume a relationship exists between nurses and the quality of care provided.
- Outcome audits determine what results, if any, occurred as a result of the nursing care provided.
- Some outcomes are influenced by aspects of care, such as the quality of medical care, the level of commitment of managerial staff, and the characteristics of the facility's policies and procedures.
- Nursing-sensitive outcomes are those that are directly affected by the quality of nursing care. Examples include client fall rates and the incidence of nosocomial infections.

Timing of audits

- Retrospective audits occur after the client receives care.
- Concurrent audits occur while the client is receiving care.
- Prospective audits predict how future client care will be affected by current level of services.

NURSE'S ROLE IN QUALITY IMPROVEMENT

- Serve as unit representative on committees developing policies and procedures.
- Use reliable resources for information (Centers for Disease Control and Prevention, professional journals, evidenced-based research). Q EBP
- Enhance knowledge and understanding of the facility's policies and procedures.
- Provide client care consistent with these policies and procedures.
- Document client care thoroughly and according to facility guidelines.
- Participate in the collection of information/data related to staff's adherence to selected policy or procedure.
- Assist with analysis of the information/data.
- Compare results with the established benchmark.
- Make a judgment about performance in regard to the findings.
- Assist with provision of education or training necessary to improve the performance of staff.
- Act as a role model by practicing in accordance with the established standard.
- Assist with re-evaluation of staff performance by collection of information/data at a specified time.

Performance appraisal, peer review, and disciplinary action

A performance appraisal is the process by which a supervisor evaluates an employee's performance in relation to the job description for that employee's position as well as other expectations the facility can have.

- Performance appraisals are done at regular intervals and can be more frequent for new employees.
- Performance expectations should be based on the standards set forth in a job description and written in objective terms.
- Performance appraisals allow nurses the opportunity to discuss personal goals with the unit manager as well as to receive feedback regarding level of performance. Performance appraisals can also be used as a motivational tool.
- Deficiencies identified during a performance appraisal or reported by coworkers might need to be addressed in a disciplinary manner.

PERFORMANCE APPRAISAL AND PEER REVIEW

- A formal system for conducting performance appraisals should be in place and used consistently. Performance appraisal tools should reflect the staff member's job description and can be based on various types of scales or surveys.
- Various sources of data should be collected to ensure an unbiased and thorough evaluation of an employee's performance.
  - Data should be collected over time and not just represent isolated incidents.
  - Actual observed behavior should be documented/used as evidence of satisfactory or unsatisfactory performance. These can be called anecdotal notes and are kept in the unit manager or equivalent position's files.
  - Peers can be a valuable source of data. Peer review is the evaluation of a colleague's practice by another peer. Peer review should:
    - Begin with an orientation of staff to the peer review process, their professional responsibility in regard to promoting growth of colleagues, and the disposition of data collected.
    - Focus on the peer's performance in relation to the job description or an appraisal tool that is based on institutional standards.
    - Be shared with the peer and usually the manager.
    - Be only part of the data used when completing a staff member's performance appraisal.
  - The employee should be given the opportunity to provide input into the evaluation.
- The unit manager should host the performance appraisal review in a private setting at a time conducive to the staff member's attendance. The unit manager should review the data with the staff member and provide the opportunity for feedback. Personal goals of the staff member are discussed and documented, including avenues for attainment. Staff members who do not agree with the unit manager's evaluation of their performance should have the opportunity to make written comments on the evaluation form and appeal the rating.

DISCIPLINARY ACTION

- Deficiencies identified during a performance appraisal or the course of employment should be presented in writing, and corrective action should be based on institutional policy regarding disciplinary actions and/or termination of employment. Evidence regarding the deficiency must support such a claim. (1.8)
- Some offenses, such as mistreatment of a client or use of alcohol or other substances while working, warrant immediate dismissal. Lesser infractions should follow a stepwise manner, giving the staff member the opportunity to correct unacceptable behavior.
- Staff members who witness an inappropriate action by a coworker should report the infraction up the chain of command. At the time of the infraction, this might be the charge nurse. The unit manager should also be notified, and written documentation by the manager is placed in the staff member's permanent file.

Conflict resolution

Conflict is the result of opposing thoughts, ideas, feelings, perceptions, behaviors, values, opinions, or actions between individuals.

- Conflict is an inevitable part of professional, social, and personal life and can have constructive or destructive results. Nurses must understand conflict and how to manage it.
- Nurses can use problem-solving and negotiation strategies to prevent a problem from evolving into a conflict. Qᴛᴄ
- Lack of conflict can create organizational stasis, while too much conflict can be demoralizing, produce anxiety, and contribute to burnout.
- Conflict can disrupt working relationships and create a stressful atmosphere.
- If conflict exists to the level that productivity and quality of care are compromised, the unit manager must attempt to identify the origin of the conflict and attempt to resolve it.

Common causes of conflict

- Ineffective communication
- Unclear expectations of team members in their various roles
- Poorly defined or actualized organizational structure
- Conflicts of interest and variance in standards
- Incompatibility of individuals
- Management or staffing changes
- Diversity related to age, gender, race, or ethnicity

CATEGORIES OF CONFLICT

INTRAPERSONAL CONFLICT

Occurs within the person and can involve internal struggle related to contradictory values or wants.

> Example: A nurse wants to move up on the career ladder but is finding that time with her family is subsequently compromised.

INTERPERSONAL CONFLICT

Occurs between two or more people with differing values, goals, or beliefs.

- Interpersonal conflict in the health care setting involves disagreement among nurses, clients, family members, and within a health care team. Bullying and incivility in the workplace are forms of interpersonal conflict.
- This is a significant issue in nursing, especially in relation to new nurses, who bring new personalities and perspectives to various health care settings.
- Interpersonal conflict contributes to burnout and work-related stress.

> Example: A new nurse is given a client assignment that is heavier than those of other nurses, and when he asks for help, it is denied.

INTERGROUP CONFLICT

Occurs between two or more groups of individuals, departments, or organizations and can be caused by a new policy or procedure, a change in leadership, or a change in organizational structure.

> Example: There is confusion as to whether it is the responsibility of the nursing unit or dietary department to pass meal trays to clients.

STAGES OF CONFLICT

Five stages of conflict exist. If the nurse manager is familiar with the stages there is an increased chance that the conflict can be resolved effectively.

STAGE 1: LATENT CONFLICT

The actual conflict has not yet developed however factors are present that have a high likelihood of causing conflict to occur.

> Example: A new scheduling policy is implemented within the organization. The nurse manager should recognize that change is a common cause of conflict.

STAGE 2: PERCEIVED CONFLICT

A party perceives that a problem is present though an actual conflict might not actually exist.

> Example: A nurse perceives that a nurse manager is unfair with scheduling. The nurse might not be aware that in reality it is only because the nurse manager misunderstood the nurse's scheduling request.

STAGE 3: FELT CONFLICT

Those involved begin to feel an emotional response to the conflict.

> Example: A nurse feels anger towards the nurse manager after finding out that she is scheduled to work two holidays in a row.

STAGE 4: MANIFEST CONFLICT

The parties involved are aware of the conflict and action is taken. Actions at this stage can be positive and strive towards conflict resolution or they can be negative and include debating, competing, or withdrawal of one or more parties from the situation.

> Example: The nurse manager and nurses on a unit agree that the current scheduling system is causing a conflict and agree to work together to come up with a solution.

STAGE 5: CONFLICT AFTERMATH

Conflict aftermath is the completion of the conflict process and can be positive or negative.

> Example: Positive conflict aftermath: the nurse manager and nurses on a unit are satisfied with the newly revised scheduling system and feel valued for being included in the conflict resolution process.

> Example: Negative conflict aftermath: the nurse manager and nurses are unable to come up with a scheduling solution that meets the needs of both parties. They agree to continue with the current system however tensions still remain increasing the risk of a recurrence of the conflict.

1.8 Steps in progressive discipline

First infraction
Informal reprimand
Manager and employee meet
Discuss the issue
Suggestions for improvement/correction

Second infraction
Written warning
Manager meets with employee to distribute written warning
Review of specific rules/policy violations
Discussion of potential consequences if infractions continue

Third infraction
Employee placed on suspension with or without pay. Time away from work gives the employee opportunity to:
Examine the issues
Consider alternatives

Fourth infraction
Employee termination
Follows after multiple warning have been given and employee continues to violate rules and policies

CONFLICT RESOLUTION STRATEGIES

PROBLEM-SOLVING

- Open communication among staff and between staff and clients can help defray the need for conflict resolution. Qᴛᴄ
- When potential sources of conflict exist, the use of open communication and problem-solving strategies are effective tools to de-escalate the situation.

Actions nurses can take to promote open communication and de-escalate conflicts

- Use "I" statements, and remember to focus on the problem, not on personal differences.
- Listen carefully to what others are saying, and try to understand their perspective.
- Move a conflict that is escalating to a private location or postpone the discussion until a later time to give everyone a chance to regain control of their emotions.
- Share ground rules with participants. For example, everyone is to be treated with respect, only one person can speak at a time, and everyone should have a chance to speak.

Steps of the problem-solving process

Identify the problem. State it in objective terms, minimizing emotional overlay.

Discuss possible solutions. Brainstorming solutions as a group can stimulate new solutions to old problems. Encourage individuals to think outside the box.

Analyze identified solutions. The potential pros and cons of each possible solution should be discussed in an attempt to narrow down the number of viable solutions.

Select a solution. Based on this analysis, select a solution for implementation.

Implement the selected solution. A procedure and time line for implementation should accompany the implementation of the selected solution.

Evaluate the solution's ability to resolve the original problem. The outcomes surrounding the new solution should be evaluated according to the predetermined time line. The solution should be given adequate time to become established as a new routine before it is evaluated. If the solution is deemed unsuccessful, the problem-solving process will need to be reinstituted and the problem discussed again.

NEGOTIATION

- Negotiation is the process by which interested parties:
  - Resolve ongoing conflicts.
  - Agree on steps to take.
  - Bargain to protect individual or collective interests.
  - Pursue outcomes that benefit mutual interests.
- Most nurses use negotiation on a daily basis.
- Negotiation can involve the use of several conflict resolution strategies.
- The focus is on a win-win solution or a win/lose-win/lose solution in which both parties win and lose a portion of their original objectives. Each party agrees to give up something and the emphasis is on accommodating differences rather than similarities between parties.

Example

One nurse offers to care for Client A today if the other will care for Client B tomorrow.

Strategy: Avoiding/Withdrawing
- Both parties know there is a conflict, but they refuse to face it or work toward a resolution.
- Can be appropriate for minor conflicts or when one party holds more power than the other party or if the issue can work itself out over time.
- Because the conflict remains, it can surface again at a later date and escalate over time.
- This is usually a lose-lose solution.

Strategy: Smoothing
- One party attempts to "smooth" another party by trying to satisfy the other party.
- Often used to preserve or maintain a peaceful work environment.
- The focus can be on what is agreed upon, leaving conflict largely unresolved.
- This is usually a lose-lose solution.

Strategy: Competing/Coercing
- One party pursues a desired solution at the expense of others.
- Managers can use this when a quick or unpopular decision must be made.
- The party who loses something can experience anger, aggravation, and a desire for retribution.
- This is usually a win-lose solution.

Strategy: Cooperating/ Accommodating
- One party sacrifices something, allowing the other party to get what it wants. This is the opposite of competing.
- The original problem might not actually be resolved.
- The solution can contribute to future conflict.
- This is a lose-win solution.

Strategy: Compromising/Negotiating
- Each party gives up something.
- To consider this a win/lose-win/lose solution, both parties must give up something equally important. If one party gives up more than the other, it can become a win-lose solution.

Strategy: Collaborating
- Both parties set aside their original individual goals work together to achieve a new common goal.
- Requires mutual respect, positive communication, and shared decision-making between parties.
- This is a win-win solution.

Example

An experienced nurse on a urology unit arrives to work on the night shift. The unit manager immediately asks the nurse to float to a pediatrics unit because the hospital census is high and they are understaffed. The nurse has always maintained a positive attitude when asked to work on another medical-surgical unit but states she does not feel comfortable in the pediatric setting. The manager insists the nurse is the most qualified.

Strategy: Avoiding/Withdrawing/Smoothing
The nurse basically cannot use these strategies due to the immediacy of the situation. The assignment cannot be simply avoided or smoothed over; it must be accepted or rejected.

Strategy: Competing/Coercing
- If the nurse truly feels unqualified to work on the pediatric unit, then this approach can be appropriate: the nurse must win and the manager must lose.
- Although risking termination by refusing the assignment, the nurse should take an assertive approach and inform the manager that pediatric clients would be placed at risk.

Strategy: Cooperating/Accommodating
- If the nurse decides to accommodate the manager's request, then the pediatric clients can be at risk for incompetent care.
- Practice liability is another issue for consideration.

Strategy: Compromising/Negotiating
- This approach generally minimizes the losses for all involved while making certain each party gains something.

  For example, the nurse might offer to work on another medical-surgical unit if someone from that unit feels comfortable in the pediatric environment.

- Although each party is giving up something (the manager gives in to a different solution and the nurse still has to work on another unit), this sort of compromise can result in a win–win resolution.

Strategy: Collaborating
Both the nurse manager and nurse come to the agreement providing safe and competent care of the children on the pediatric unit is the common goal. While they might need to compromise/negotiate to address the immediate need they can collaborate to achieve a solution that avoids this situation in the future.

  For example, the nurse might agree to orient to the pediatric unit in order to become competent for future assignments and the nurse manager can enlist the services of a staffing agency that provides pediatric nurses on an as needed basis.

ASSERTIVE COMMUNICATION

- Use of assertive communication can be necessary during conflict negotiation.
- Assertive communication allows expression in direct, honest, and nonthreatening ways that do not infringe upon the rights of others.
- It is a communication style that acknowledges and deals with conflict, recognizes others as equals, and provides a direct statement of feelings.

Elements of assertive communication

- Selecting an appropriate location for verbal exchange
- Maintenance of eye contact
- Establishing trust
- Being sensitive to cultural needs
- Speaking using "I" statements and including affective elements of the situation
- Avoiding "you" statements that can indicate blame
- Stating concerns using open, honest, direct statements
- Conveying empathy
- Focusing on the behavior or issue of conflict and avoiding personal attacks
- Concluding with a statement that describes a fair solution

GRIEVANCES

- A grievance is a wrong perceived by an employee based on a feeling of unfair treatment that is considered grounds for a formal complaint.
- Grievances that cannot be satisfactorily resolved between the parties involved can require management by a third party.
- Facilities have a formal grievance policy that should be followed when a conflict cannot be resolved.
- The steps of an institution's grievance procedure should be outlined in the grievance policy.

Typical steps of the grievance process

- Formal presentation of the complaint using the proper chain of command
- Formal hearing if the issue is not resolved at a lower level
- Professional mediation if a solution is not reached during a formal hearing

Resource management

Resource management includes budgeting and resource allocation. Human, financial, and material resources must be considered.

- Budgeting is usually the responsibility of the unit manager, but staff nurses can be asked to provide input.
- Resource allocation is a responsibility of the unit manager as well as every practicing nurse.
- Providing cost-effective client care should not compromise quality of care.

Resources (supplies, equipment, personnel) are critical to accomplishing the goals and objectives of a health care facility, so it is essential for nurses to understand how to effectively manage resources. Qᵍⁱ

COST-EFFECTIVE CARE

Cost-containment

Strategies that promote efficient and competent client care while also producing needed revenues for the continued productivity of the organization

> Example: The use of managed care strives to provide clients with a plan designed to meet the needs of their individual medical problem while eliminating the unnecessary use of resources or extended hospital stays.

Cost-effective

Strategies that achieve optimal results in relation to the money spent to achieve those results. In other words cost-effective means "getting your money's worth."

> Example: Spending increased money on staff training for transmission-based precautions resulting in the increased and effective use of PPE for client care. These actions have the end result of a decrease in infection transmission and an overall savings in the cost of caring for clients who would have acquired these infections.

COST-EFFECTIVE CARE STRATEGIES

Providing clients with needed education to decrease or eliminate future medical costs associated with future complications.

> Example: Teaching a client who has a new diagnosis of diabetes mellitus how to adjust the dosage of insulin depending on activity level reducing the risk of hypoglycemia resulting in the need for medical care.

Promoting the use of evidence-based care resulting in improved client care outcomes.

> Example: Implementing the use of evidence-based techniques to care for clients who have indwelling catheters resulting in a decreased incidence of catheter-acquired urinary tract infections.

Promoting cost-effective resource management.

> Example: Using all levels of personnel to their fullest when making assignments. Delegating effectively to members of the nursing care team.

> Example: Providing necessary equipment and properly charging clients.

> Example: Returning uncontaminated, unused equipment to the appropriate department for credit.

> Example: Using equipment properly to prevent wastage.

> Example: Providing training to staff unfamiliar with equipment.

> Example: Returning equipment (IV pumps) to the proper department (central service, central distribution) as soon as it is no longer needed. This action will prevent further cost to clients.

Application Exercises

1. A nurse enters the room of a client who is on contact precautions and finds the client lying on the floor. Which of the following actions should the nurse take first?

   A. Call the provider.

   B. Ask a staff member for assistance getting the client back in bed.

   C. Inspect the client for injuries.

   D. Instruct the client to ask for help if he needs to get out of bed.

2. An RN on a medical-surgical unit is making assignments at the beginning of the shift. Which of the following tasks should the nurse delegate to the PN?

   A. Obtain vital signs for a client who is 2 hr postprocedure following a cardiac catheterization.

   B. Administer a unit of packed red blood cells (RBCs) to a client who has cancer.

   C. Instruct a client who is scheduled for discharge in the performance of wound care.

   D. Develop a plan of care for a newly admitted client who has pneumonia.

3. A PN ending her shift reports to the RN that a newly hired AP has not calculated the intake and output for several clients. Which of the following actions should the RN take?

   A. Complete an incident report.

   B. Delegate this task to the PN.

   C. Ask the AP if she needs assistance.

   D. Notify the nurse manager.

4. A nurse manager is developing an orientation plan for newly licensed nurses. Which of the following information should the manager include in the plan? (Select all that apply.)

   A. Skill proficiency

   B. Assignment to a preceptor

   C. Budgetary principles

   D. Computerized charting

   E. Socialization into unit culture

   F. Facility policies and procedures

5. A nurse manager is providing information about the audit process to members of the nursing team. Which of the following information should the nurse manager include? (Select all that apply.)

   A. A structure audit evaluates the setting and resources available to provide care.

   B. An outcome audit evaluates the results of the nursing care provided.

   C. A root cause analysis is indicated when a sentinel event occurs.

   D. Retrospective audits are conducted while the client is receiving care.

   E. After data collection is completed, it is compared to a benchmark.

6. A nurse is participating in a quality improvement study of a procedure frequently performed on the unit. Which of the following information will provide data regarding the efficacy of the procedure?

   A. Frequency with which procedure is performed

   B. Client satisfaction with performance of procedure

   C. Incidence of complications related to procedure

   D. Accurate documentation of how procedure was performed

7. A nurse is hired to replace a staff member who has resigned. After working on the unit for several weeks, the nurse notices that the unit manager does not intervene when there is conflict between team members, even when it escalates. Which of the following conflict resolution strategies is the unit manager demonstrating?

   A. Avoidance

   B. Smoothing

   C. Cooperating

   D. Negotiating

Application Exercises Key

1. A. The nurse should notify the provider to determine whether the client needs further examination and treatment, but there is another action the nurse should take first.

   B. The nurse should seek assistance in returning the client to bed to prevent further harm to the client, but there is another action the nurse should take first.

   C. **CORRECT:** The first action the nurse should take using the nursing process is to assess the client.

   D. The nurse should instruct the client to ask for help if he needs to get out of bed to help prevent future falls, but there is another action the nurse should take first.

   Ⓝ *NCLEX® Connection: Management of Care, Establishing Priorities*

2. A. **CORRECT:** It is within the scope of practice of the PN to monitor a client who is 2 hr postprocedure for a cardiac catheterization.

   B. The RN is responsible for administering blood components including packed RBCs because this outside of the scope of practice for the PN.

   C. The RN is responsible for client education. It is within the scope of practice of the PN to reinforce but not provide initial client education.

   D. The RN is responsible for developing a plan of care for a client. It is within the scope of practice for the PN to suggest additions to but not develop the plan of care.

   Ⓝ *NCLEX® Connection: Management of Care, Assignment, Delegation and Supervision*

3. A. An incident report is indicated when a critical incident has occurred. It is not necessary to complete an incident report in this situation.

   B. The nurse should not redelegate a task.

   C. **CORRECT:** The nurse should find out what the AP knows about performing the task and provide education for the AP if indicated.

   D. The RN is capable of handling the situation. It is not necessary to notify the nurse manager.

   Ⓝ *NCLEX® Connection: Management of Care, Assignment, Delegation and Supervision*

4. A. **CORRECT:** The purpose of orientation is to assist the newly licensed nurse to transition from the role of student to the role of employee and licensed nurse. The nurse manager should include evaluation of skill proficiency and provide additional instruction as indicated.

   B. **CORRECT:** The purpose of orientation is to assist the newly licensed nurse to transition from the role of student to the role of employee and licensed nurse. The nurse manager should include assignment of a preceptor to ease the transition of the newly licensed nurse.

   C. Budgetary principles are an administrative skill that is usually the responsibility of the unit manager.

   D. **CORRECT:** The purpose of orientation is to assist the newly licensed nurse to transition from the role of student to the role of employee and licensed nurse. The nurse manager should include computerized charting, which is an essential skill for the newly licensed nurse.

   E. **CORRECT:** The purpose of orientation is to assist the newly licensed nurse to transition from the role of student to the role of employee and licensed nurse. The nurse manager should include socialization to the unit as a way to ease the transition of the newly licensed nurse.

   F. **CORRECT:** The purpose of orientation is to assist the newly licensed nurse to transition from the role of student to the role of employee and licensed nurse. The nurse manager should include information about facility policies and procedures, which is essential information for the newly licensed nurse.

   Ⓝ *NCLEX® Connection: Management of Care, Concepts of Management*

5. A. **CORRECT:** A structure audit evaluates the setting in which care is provided and includes resources such as equipment and staffing levels.

   B. **CORRECT:** An outcome audit evaluates the effectiveness of nursing care. It should include observable data, such as infection rates among clients.

   C. **CORRECT:** A root cause analysis is indicated when a sentinel event occurs. A sentinel event is a serious problem such as injury to or death of a client. Immediate investigation of the problem is indicated. The health care team can use root cause analysis to study the problem and take measures to prevent reoccurrence.

   D. Retrospective audits are conducted when the client is no longer receiving care.

   E. **CORRECT:** The benchmark is set at the beginning of the process and then it is compared to the data after collection is completed.

   Ⓝ *NCLEX® Connection: Management of Care, Performance Improvement (Quality Improvement)*

6. A. The frequency with which the procedure is performed is important. The team can take the frequency in which the procedure is performed under consideration in the planning process, but this information does not address the efficacy of the procedure.

   B. The team should take client satisfaction under consideration in the planning process, but this information does not address the efficacy of the procedure.

   C. **CORRECT:** The incidence of complications related to the procedure is an outcome measure directly related to the efficacy of the procedure.

   D. The team can take accuracy of documentation under consideration in the planning process, but this information does not address the efficacy of the procedure.

   Ⓝ *NCLEX® Connection: Management of Care, Performance Improvement (Quality Improvement)*

7. A. **CORRECT:** The goal in resolving conflict is a win-win situation. The unit manager is using an ineffective strategy, avoidance, to deal with this conflict. She is aware of the conflict but is not attempting to resolve it.

   B. The goal in resolving conflict is a win-win solution. When smoothing is used, one person attempts to "smooth" the other party and/or point out areas in which the parties agree. This is typically a lose-lose solution.

   C. The goal in resolving a conflict is a win-win solution. When cooperating is used, one party allows the other party to win. This is a lose-win solution.

   D. The goal in resolving a conflict is a win-win solution. When negotiating is used, each party gives up something. If one party gives up more than the other, this can become a win-lose solution.

   Ⓝ *NCLEX® Connection: Management of Care, Concepts of Management*

ℕ NCLEX® Connections

When reviewing the following chapter, keep in mind the relevant topics and tasks of the NCLEX outline, in particular:

Client Needs: Management of Care

CASE MANAGEMENT: Explore resources available to assist the client with achieving or maintaining independence.

COLLABORATION WITH INTERDISCIPLINARY TEAM
Review plan of care to ensure continuity across disciplines.

Identify significant information to report to other disciplines.

CONCEPTS OF MANAGEMENT: Act as liaison between the client and others.

CONTINUITY OF CARE: Use documents to record and communicate client information.

REFERRALS: Identify community resources for the client.

Coordinating Client Care

One of the primary roles of nursing is the coordination and management of client care in collaboration with the health care team. In so doing, high-quality health care is provided as clients move through the health care system in a cost-effective and time-efficient manner. Qᴛᴄ

To effectively coordinate client care, a nurse must have an understanding of collaboration with the interprofessional team, principles of case management, continuity of care (including consultations, referrals, transfers, and discharge planning), and motivational principles to encourage and empower self, staff, colleagues, and other members of the interprofessional team.

COLLABORATION WITH THE INTERPROFESSIONAL TEAM

An interprofessional team is a group of health care professionals from various disciplines. Collaboration involves discussion of client care issues in making health care decisions, especially for clients who have multiple problems. The specialized knowledge and skills of each discipline are used in the development of an interprofessional plan of care that addresses multiple problems. Nurses should recognize that the collaborative efforts of the interprofessional team allow the achievement of results that a team member would be incapable of accomplishing alone.

- Nurse-provider collaboration should be fostered to create a climate of mutual respect and collaborative practice.
- Collaboration occurs among different levels of nurses and nurses with different areas of expertise.
- Collaboration should also occur between the interprofessional team, the client, and the client's family/significant others when an interprofessional plan of care is being developed.
- Collaboration is a form of conflict resolution that results in a win-win solution for both the client and health care team.

NURSE QUALITIES FOR EFFECTIVE COLLABORATION

- Good communication skills
- Assertiveness
- Conflict negotiation skills
- Leadership skills
- Professional presence
- Decision-making and critical thinking

THE NURSE'S ROLE

- Coordinate the interprofessional team.
- Have a holistic understanding of the client, the client's health care needs, and the health care system.
- Provide the opportunity for care to be provided with continuity over time and across disciplines.
- Provide the client with the opportunity to be a partner in the development of the plan of care.
- Provide information during rounds and interprofessional team meetings regarding the status of the client's health.
- Provide an avenue for the initiation of a consultation related to a specific health care issue.
- Provide a link to postdischarge resources that might need a referral.

VARIABLES THAT AFFECT COLLABORATION

Decision-making styles

The interprofessional team within a facility is challenged with making sound decisions about how client care is delivered. A variety of decision-making styles are available for use depending upon the needs of the situation. Often the group leader decides the decision-making style the team will use. Decision-making styles vary in regard to the amount of data collected and the number of options generated.

DECISIVE: The team uses a minimum amount of data and generates one option.

FLEXIBLE: The team uses a limited amount of data and generates several options.

HIERARCHICAL: The team uses a large amount of data and generates one option.

INTEGRATIVE: The team uses a large amount of data and generates several options.

Hierarchical influence on decision-making

Decision-making is also influenced by the facility hierarchy. In a centralized hierarchy, nurses at the top of the organizational chart make most of the decisions. In a decentralized hierarchy, staff nurses who provide direct client care are included in the decision-making process. Large organizations benefit from the use of decentralized decision-making because managers at the top of the hierarchy do not have firsthand knowledge of unit-level challenges or problems. Decentralized decision-making promotes job satisfaction among staff nurses.

Behavioral change strategies

Although bombarded with constant change, members of the interprofessional team can be resistant to change. Three strategies a manager can use to promote change are the rational-empirical, normative-reeducative and the power-coercive. Often the manager uses a combination of these strategies.

RATIONAL-EMPIRICAL: The manager provides factual information to support the change. Used when resistance to change is minimal.

NORMATIVE-REEDUCATIVE: The manager focuses on interpersonal relationships to promote change.

POWER-COERCIVE: The manager uses rewards to promote change. Used when individuals are highly resistant to change.

Stages of team formation

Teams typically work through a group formation process before reaching peak performance.

FORMING: Members of the team get to know each other. The leader defines tasks for the team and offers direction.

STORMING: Conflict arises, and team members begin to express polarized views. The team establishes rules, and members begin to take on various roles.

NORMING: The team establishes rules. Members show respect for one another and begin to accomplish some of the tasks.

PERFORMING: The team focuses on accomplishment of tasks.

Generational differences team members

Generational differences influence the value system of the members of an interprofessional team and can affect how members function within the team. Generational differences can be challenging for members of a team, but working with individuals from different generations also can bring strength to the team. **(2.1)**

MAGNET RECOGNITION PROGRAM

The interprofessional team is charged with maintaining continuous quality improvement. The nursing staff can choose to demonstrate quality nursing care by seeking Magnet Recognition.

- The American Nurses Credentialing Center awards Magnet Recognition to health care facilities that provide high-quality client care and attract and retain well-qualified nurses. The term magnet is used to recognize the facility's power to draw nurses to the facility and to retain them.
- Fourteen forces of magnetism provide the framework for the magnet review process. The first step for a facility that applies for magnet recognition is to complete a self-appraisal based on a set of established standards. It is important that all levels of nursing participate in the application process.
- After documentation that the standards have been met, an on-site appraisal is conducted. A facility that meets the standards is awarded magnet status for a four-year period.
- To maintain magnet status, the facility must maintain the established standards and submit an annual report.

2.1 Generational characteristics

	VETERAN	BABY BOOMER	GENERATION X	GENERATION Y
BIRTH YEAR	1925-1942	1943-1960	1961-1980	1981-2000
CHARACTERISTICS	Supports the status quo Accepts authority Appreciates hierarchy Loyal to employer	Accepts authority Workaholics Some struggle with new technology Loyal to employer	Adapts easily to change Personal life and family are important Proficient with technology Makes frequent job changes	Optimistic and self-confident Values achievement Technology is a way of life At ease with cultural diversity

CASE MANAGEMENT

Case management is the coordination of care provided by an interprofessional team from the time a client starts receiving care until she no longer receives services. Q_{TC}

PRINCIPLES OF CASE MANAGEMENT

- Case management focuses on managed care of the client through collaboration of the health care team in acute and postacute settings.
- The goal of case management is to avoid fragmentation of care and control cost.
- A case manager collaborates with the interprofessional health care team during the assessment of a client's needs and subsequent care planning, and follows up by monitoring the achievement of desired client outcomes within established time parameters.
- A case manager can be a nurse, social worker, or other designated health care professional. A case manager's role and knowledge expectations are extensive. Therefore, case managers are required to have advanced practice degrees or advanced training in this area.
- Case manager nurses do not usually provide direct client care.
- Case managers usually oversee a caseload of clients who have similar disorders or treatment regimens.
- Case managers in the community coordinate resources and services for clients whose care is based in a residential setting.
- A critical or clinical pathway or care map can be used to support the implementation of clinical guidelines and protocols. These tools are usually based on cost and length of stay parameters mandated by prospective payment systems such as Medicare and insurance companies.

NURSING ROLE IN CASE MANAGEMENT

- Coordinating care, particularly for clients who have complex health care needs
- Facilitating continuity of care
- Improving efficiency of care and utilization of resources
- Enhancing quality of care provided
- Limiting unnecessary costs and lengthy stays
- Advocating for the client and family

CONTINUITY OF CARE: CONSULTATIONS, REFERRALS, TRANSFERS, AND DISCHARGE PLANNING

Continuity of care refers to the consistency of care provided as clients move through the health care system. It enhances the quality of client care and facilitates the achievement of positive client outcomes. Q_{PCC}

- Continuity of care is desired as clients move from one:
  - Level of care to another, such as from the ICU to a medical unit
  - Facility to another, such as from an acute care facility to a skilled facility
  - Unit/department to another, such as from the PACU to the postsurgical unit
- Nurses are responsible for facilitating continuity of care and coordinating care through documentation, reporting, and collaboration.
- A formal, written plan of care enhances coordination of care between nurses, interprofessional team members, and providers.

NURSING ROLE IN CONTINUITY OF CARE

The nurse's role as coordinator of care includes the following.
- Facilitating the continuity of care provided by members of the health care team.
- Acting as a representative of the client and as a liaison when collaborating with the provider and other members of the health care team. When acting as a liaison, the nurse serves in the role of client advocate by protecting the rights of clients and ensuring that client needs are met.

As the coordinator of care, the nurse is responsible for:
- Admission, transfer, discharge, and postdischarge prescriptions.
- Initiation, revision, and evaluation of the plan of care.
- Reporting the client's status to other nurses and the provider.
- Coordinating the discharge plan.
- Facilitating referrals and the use of community resources.

DOCUMENTATION

Documentation to facilitate continuity of care includes the following.
- Graphic records that illustrate trending of assessment data such as vital signs
- Flow sheets that reflect routine care completed and other care-related data
- Nurses' notes that describe changes in client status or unusual circumstances
- Client care summaries that serve as quick references for client care information
- Nursing care plans that set the standard for care provided.
  - Standardized nursing care plans provide a starting point for the nurse responsible for care plan development.
  - Standardized plans must be individualized to each client.
  - All documentation should reflect the plan of care.

COMMUNICATION AND CONTINUITY OF CARE

Communication tools
- Poor communication can lead to adverse outcomes, including sentinel events (unexpected death or serious injury of a client).
- A number of communication hand-off tools are available to improve communication and promote client safety: I-SBAR, PACE, I PASS the BATON, Five P's Qs

Change-of-shift report
- Performed with the nurse who is assuming responsibility for the client's care.
- Describes the current health status of the client.
- Informs the next shift of pertinent client care information.
- Provides the oncoming nurse the opportunity to ask questions and clarify the plan of care.
- Should be given in a private area, such as a conference room or at the bedside, to protect client confidentiality.

Report to the provider QTC
- Assessment data integral to changes in client status
- Recommendations for changes in the plan of care
- Clarification of prescriptions

CONSULTATIONS

- A consultant is a professional who provides expert advice in a particular area. A consultation is requested to help determine what treatment/services the client requires. QPCC
- Consultants provide expertise for clients who require a specific type of knowledge or service (a cardiologist for a client who had a myocardial infarction, a psychiatrist for a client whose risk for suicide must be assessed).

The nurse's role regarding consultations
- Initiate necessary consults or notify the provider of the client's needs so the consult can be initiated.
- Provide the consultant with all pertinent information about the problem (information from the client/family, the client's medical records).
- Incorporate the consultant's recommendations into the client's plan of care.

REFERRALS

A referral is a formal request for a service by another care provider. It is made so that the client can access the care identified by the provider or the consultant. QPCC
- The care can be provided in the acute setting or outside the facility.
- Clients being discharged from health care facilities to their home can still require nursing care.
- Discharge referrals are based on client needs in relation to actual and potential problems and can be facilitated with the assistance of social services, especially if there is a need for:
  - Specialized equipment (cane, walker, wheelchair, grab bars in bathroom)
  - Specialized therapists (physical, occupational, speech)
  - Care providers (home health nurse, hospice nurse, home health aide)
- Knowledge of community and online resources is necessary to appropriately link the client with needed services.

The nurse's role regarding referrals
- Begin discharge planning upon the client's admission.
- Evaluate client/family competencies in relation to home care prior to discharge.
- Involve the client and family in care planning.
- Collaborate with other health care professionals to ensure all health care needs are met and necessary referrals are made.
- Complete referral forms to ensure proper reimbursement for prescribed services.

TRANSFERS

Clients can be transferred from one unit, department, or one facility to another. Continuity of care must be maintained as the client moves from one setting to another.

- The use of communication hand-off tools (I PASS the BATON, PACE) promotes continuity of care and client safety. Qs
- The nurse's role regarding transfers is to provide written and verbal report of the client's status and care needs.
  - Client medical diagnosis and care providers
  - Client demographic information
  - Overview of health status, plan of care, and recent progress
  - Alterations that can precipitate an immediate concern
  - Most recent vital signs and medications, including when a PRN was given
  - Notification of assessments or client care needed within the next few hours
  - Allergies
  - Diet and activity prescriptions
  - Presence of or need for specific equipment or adaptive devices (oxygen, suction, wheelchair)
  - Advance directives and whether a client is to be resuscitated in the event of cardiac or respiratory arrest
  - Family involvement in care and health care proxy, if applicable

DISCHARGE PLANNING

Discharge planning is an interprofessional process that is started by the nurse at the time of the client's admission. Qtc

- The nurse conducts discharge planning with both the client and client's family for optimal results.
- Discharge planning serves as a starting point for continuity of care. As client care needs are identified, measures can be taken to prepare for the provision of needed support.
- The need for additional services such as home health, physical therapy, and respite care can be addressed before the client is discharged so the service is in place when the client arrives home.
- A client who leaves a facility without a prescription for discharge from the provider is considered leaving against medical advice (AMA). A client who is legally competent has the legal right to leave the facility at any time. The nurse should immediately notify the provider. If the client is at risk for harm, it is imperative that the nurse explain the risk involved in leaving the facility. The individual should sign a form relinquishing responsibility for any complications that arise from discontinuing prescribed care. The nurse should document all communication, as well as the specific advice that was provided for the client. A nurse who tries to prevent the client from leaving the facility can face legal charges of assault, battery, and false imprisonment.

Discharge instructions

- Step-by-step instructions for procedures to be done at home. Clients should be given the opportunity to provide a return demonstration of these procedures to validate learning.
- Medication regimen instructions for home, including adverse effects and actions to take to minimize them.
- Precautions to take when performing procedures or administering medications.
- Indications of medication adverse effects or medical complications that the client should report to the provider.
- Names and numbers of providers and community services the client or family can contact.
- Plans for follow-up care and therapies.

The nurse's role with regard to discharge is to provide a written summary including:

- Type of discharge (prescribed by provider, AMA).
- Date and time of discharge, who accompanied the client, and how the client was transported (wheelchair to a private car, stretcher to an ambulance).
- Discharge destination (home, long-term care facility).
- A summary of the client's condition at discharge (gait, dietary intake, use of assistive devices, blood glucose).
- A description of any unresolved problems and plans for follow-up.
- Disposition of valuables, medications brought from home, and prescriptions.
- A copy of the client's discharge instructions.

INTERFACILITY TRANSFER FORM

_____

_____

	Place label here

_____

TRANSFER FROM: _____

Client Condition: _____ Stable _____ Unstable

Reason for transfer and Benefits and Risks of transfer:
____ Client/responsible person's request
____ Need for higher level of care not available at this facility
____ Need for diagnostic equipment not available at this facility
____ Transfer request by:
_____, MD
____ Other: _____

Benefits of Transfer:
_____
_____

Risks of Transfer:
____ Death
____ Vehicular accident
____ Bleeding
____ Pulmonary Decompensation
____ Cardiac Decompensation
____ Delivery in route
____ Deterioration of medical condition:

_____
____ Additional delay in receiving appropriate treatment
____ Other _____
____ I certify that based upon the information available at the time of transfer, the medical benefits and treatment at the accepting facility, outweigh the increased risks to the client in the case of pregnancy, the unborn infant.
____ After client assessment, I certify that I have discussed the risks and benefits to the client that were known to me at the time of transfer.
____ Medical Diagnosis:
_____
_____

Provider's Name: _____

Signature: _____
Date: _____ **Time:** _____

I acknowledge by my signature that I agree to my transfer to the receiving facility and the transferring provider has discussed with me the risks and benefits of transfer.

Client Signature:
_____

Client unable to sign, Signature of Responsible person:
_____
Relationship: _____

Approval of Transfer
____ The receiving facility has agreed to accept the client, provide appropriate medical treatment and has available and qualified personnel for the treatment of this client.

_____

Name/title of transferring facility contact receiving above approval:
_____

Name/title of receiving facility contact granting above approval:
_____

Name of receiving facility: _____
Name of provider receiving client from transferring provider:
_____

Name of transferring nursing personnel giving report:
_____

Name of receiving nursing personnel receiving report:
_____

Available space confirmed by: _____ Time: _____

Method of Transfer
Name of transferring facility: _____
Time of arrival: _____ Time of transfer: _____
Qualified personnel with appropriate medical equipment which will be able to use all necessary and appropriate life support measures will transfer the client:
_____ BLS _____ ALS _____ Air Transport
Other: _____

Treatment
____ The transferring facility has within its capacity provided medical treatment to minimize the risk to the client's health (and in the case of pregnancy, the unborn infant).
Treatment rendered included:
____ IV: _____
____ Medications: _____
____ Oxygen: _____
____ Procedures: _____

Vital signs at the time of transfer:
T _____ P _____ R _____ BP _____
Records sent with client:
____ Laboratory findings: _____
____ Radiographs: _____
____ EKG   Valuables
____ Medical record   ____ To the family

Discharge client assessment: _____
_____

Name of Transferring Nurse: _____
Date: _____ **Signature:** _____

Transfer Report

Name:		Birth date:	
Admission date:		Medical Record #:	
Transfer date:		Attending provider:	
Transfer from:		Address:	
Transfer to:		Phone:	
Contact: Address: Phone: Relationship:		Notify	☐ Yes ☐ No

Reason for transfer		ADLs	No assistance needed	Assistance/ supervision	Total care
Vital signs:		Walking			
T _____ P _____ R _____ BP _____ WT _____		Transfers			
Diagnosis:		Bathing			
Prognosis/rehab potential:		Eating			
Allergies:		Oral hygiene			
Diet:		Dressing			
Activity level:					
Precautions:					
Medication:	Date/time of last dose:	Prosthesis: Hearing: Speech: Vision:			
		Bowel/bladder:			
Treatment:	date/time:	Mental status: Emotional status: Additional information:			
Provider signature: Date:		Nurse signature: Date:			

Discharge Summary

ati.

Date:

Medication (include drug, route of administration, and instructions)	Route/schedule	Instructions/side effects
1.		
2.		
3.		
4.		
5.		
6.		
7.		
8.		
9.		
10.		

Treatments/procedures:

Activity:

Problems to report to provider: (list signs/symptoms pertinent to client diagnosis)

Diet:

Follow-up:

Referrals:

Personal belongings given to:

☐ Dentures　　☐ Hearing aid　　☐ Glasses/contacts

Verbalizes understanding of present physical condition?	☐ Yes	☐ No
Verbalizes understanding of discharge instructions?	☐ Yes	☐ No

The above discharge instructions have been explained and a copy has been provided to me

　　　　　　　　　　　　　　　　　　　　Client/significant other

Mode of transport:　　　　　　　　Discharged via: ☐ stretcher, ☐ amb., ☐ w/c

Accompanied by:

Destination:　　　　　　With whom:　　　　　　Departure time:

Nurse's signature:

Application Exercises

1. A nurse is preparing to transfer an older adult client who is 72 hr postoperative to a long-term care facility. Which of the following information should the nurse include in the transfer report? (Select all that apply).

   A. Type of anesthesia used

   B. Advance directives status

   C. Vital signs on day of admission

   D. Medical diagnosis

   E. Need for specific equipment

2. A nurse is participating in an interprofessional conference for a client who has a recent C6 spinal cord injury. The client worked as a construction worker prior to his injury. Which of the following members of the interprofessional team should participate in planning care for this client? (Select all that apply.)

   A. Physical therapist

   B. Speech therapist

   C. Occupational therapist

   D. Psychologist

   E. Vocational counselor

3. A nurse manager is working with a committee of nurses to update policies for new employee orientation. The nurse manager directs the team to collect as much data as possible and recommend several options. Which of the following decision-making styles is the nurse manager demonstrating?

   A. Decisive

   B. Flexible

   C. Hierarchical

   D. Integrative

4. A nurse who has just assumed the role of unit manager is examining her skills in interprofessional collaboration. Which of the following actions support the nurse's interprofessional collaboration? (Select all that apply.)

   A. Use aggressive communication when addressing the team.

   B. Recognize the knowledge and skills of each member of the team.

   C. Ensure that a nurse is assigned to serve as the group facilitator for all interprofessional meetings.

   D. Encourage the client and family to participate in the team meeting.

   E. Support team member requests for referral.

5. A nurse on a telemetry unit is caring for a client who was admitted 2 hr ago and has chest pain. The client becomes angry and tells the nurse that there is nothing wrong with him and that he is going home immediately. Which of the following actions should the nurse take? (Select all that apply.)

   A. Notify the client's family of his intent to leave the facility. .

   B. Document that the client left the facility against medical advice (AMA).

   C. Explain to the client the risks involved if he chooses to leave.

   D. Ask the client to sign a form relinquishing responsibility of the facility.

   E. Prevent the client from leaving the facility until the provider arrives.

PRACTICE Active Learning Scenario

A nurse is explaining her role as case manager to a newly licensed nurse. What should the case manager include in her discussion? Use the ATI Active Learning Template: Basic Concept to complete this item.

UNDERLYING PRINCIPLES: Identify three roles of a case manager.

Application Exercises Key

1. A. The nurse should include only information that is pertinent to the transfer. The receiving nurse and facility do not need to know the type of anesthesia used in order to provide care or address the client's current needs.

    B. **CORRECT:** The receiving nurse and facility need to know advance directive status in order to provide care and address the client's current needs.

    C. The receiving nurse and facility do not need to know admission vital signs in order to provide care or address the client's current needs. However, the nurse should provide the most recent set of vital signs in the report.

    D. **CORRECT:** The receiving nurse and facility need to know the client's medical diagnosis in order to provide care and address the client's current needs.

    E. **CORRECT:** The receiving nurse and facility need to know the client's need for specific equipment in order to provide care and address the client's current needs.

    Ⓝ *NCLEX® Connection: Management of Care, Continuity of Care*

2. A. **CORRECT:** The client will need the assistance of a physical therapist to assist with mobility skills and maintain muscle strength.

    B. A speech therapist assists a client who has speech and swallowing problems, which are not anticipated for this client.

    C. **CORRECT:** The client will need the assistance of an occupational therapist to learn how to perform activities of daily living.

    D. **CORRECT:** The client will need the assistance of a psychologist to adapt to the psychosocial impact of the injury.

    E. **CORRECT:** The client will need the assistance of a vocational counselor to explore options for re-employment.

    Ⓝ *NCLEX® Connection: Management of Care, Collaboration with Interdisciplinary Team*

3. A. When the decisive decision-making style is used, the team uses a minimum amount of data and generates one option.

    B. When the flexible decision-making style is used, the team uses a limited amount of data and generates several options.

    C. When the hierarchical decision-making style is used, the team uses a large amount of data and generates one option.

    D. **CORRECT:** When the integrative decision-making style is used, the team uses a large amount of data and generates several options.

    Ⓝ *NCLEX® Connection: Management of Care, Concepts of Management*

4. A. The nurse should use assertive skills when communicating with the interprofessional team.

    B. **CORRECT:** The nurse should recognize that each member of the team has specific skills to contribute to the collaboration process.

    C. A nurse can serve as the facilitator. However, this role can be assumed by any member of the team.

    D. **CORRECT:** Collaboration should occur among the client, family, and interprofessional team.

    E. **CORRECT:** The nurse should support suggestions for referrals to link clients to appropriate resources.

    Ⓝ *NCLEX® Connection: Management of Care, Collaboration with Interdisciplinary Team*

5. A. The client has the legal right to leave the hospital against medical advice. Notifying the client's family without the client's permission violates the client's right to confidentiality.

    B. **CORRECT:** When documenting a discharge, the nurse should document the type of discharge, including an AMA discharge.

    C. **CORRECT:** The nurse is legally responsible to warn the client of the risks involved in leaving the hospital against medical advice.

    D. **CORRECT:** Clients who leave the hospital prior to a prescribed discharge are asked to sign a form to provide legal protection for the hospital.

    E. A nurse who tries to prevent a client from leaving the hospital by any action, such as threatening him or refusing to give him his clothes, can be charged with assault, battery, and false imprisonment.

    Ⓝ *NCLEX® Connection: Management of Care, Client Rights*

PRACTICE Answer

Using ATI Active Learning Template: Basic Concept

UNDERLYING PRINCIPLES: Roles of a case manager
- Coordinating care of clients who have complex health care needs
- Facilitating continuity of care
- Improving efficiency of care
- Enhancing quality of care provided
- Limiting cost and lengthy stays
- Advocating for the client and family

Ⓝ *NCLEX® Connection: Management of Care, Concepts of Management*

NCLEX® Connections

When reviewing the following chapter, keep in mind the relevant topics and tasks of the NCLEX outline, in particular:

Client Needs: Management of Care

ADVANCE DIRECTIVES/SELF-DETERMINATION/LIFE PLANNING: Integrate advance directives into client plan of care.

ADVOCACY: Discuss identified treatment options with client and respect their decisions.

CLIENT RIGHTS: Provide education to clients and staff about client rights and responsibilities.

CONFIDENTIALITY/INFORMATION SECURITY: Assess staff member and client understanding of confidentiality requirements.

ETHICAL PRACTICE: Recognize ethical dilemmas and take appropriate action.

INFORMED CONSENT: Verify that the client received appropriate procedure education and consents to care and procedures.

INFORMATION TECHNOLOGY: Apply knowledge of facility regulations when accessing client records.

LEGAL RIGHTS AND RESPONSIBILITIES: Educate the client/staff on legal issues.

CHAPTER 3 *Professional Responsibilities*

Professional responsibilities are the obligations that nurses have to their clients. To meet their professional responsibilities, nurses must be knowledgeable in the following areas: client rights, advocacy, informed consent, advance directives, confidentiality and information security, information technology, legal practice, disruptive behavior, and ethical practice.

Client rights

- Client rights are the legal guarantees that clients have with regard to their health care.
  - Clients using the services of a health care institution retain their rights as individuals and citizens of the United States. The American Hospital Association (AHA) identifies client rights in health care settings in the Patient Care Partnership (www.aha.org).
  - Residents in nursing facilities that participate in Medicare programs similarly retain resident rights under statutes that govern the operation of these facilities.
- Nurses are accountable for protecting the rights of clients. Situations that require particular attention include informed consent, refusal of treatment, advance directives, confidentiality, and information security.

NURSING ROLE IN CLIENT RIGHTS

- Nurses must ensure that clients understand their rights. Nurses also must protect clients' rights during nursing care. Q𝗣𝗖𝗖
- Regardless of the client's age, nursing needs, or the setting in which care is provided, the basic tenants are the same. Each client has the right to the following.
  - Be informed about all aspects of care and take an active role in the decision-making process.
  - Accept, refuse, or request modification to the plan of care.
  - Receive care that is delivered by competent individuals who treat the client with respect.

REFUSAL OF TREATMENT

The Patient Self-Determination Act (PSDA) stipulates that on admission to a health care facility, all clients must be informed of their right to accept or refuse care. Competent adults have the right to refuse treatment, including the right to leave a health care facility without a prescription for discharge from the provider.

- If the client refuses a treatment or procedure, the client is asked to sign a document indicating that he understands the risk involved with refusing the treatment or procedure, and that he has chosen to refuse it.
- When a client decides to leave the facility without a prescription for discharge, the nurse notifies the provider and discusses with the client the potential risks associated with leaving the facility prior to discharge.
- The nurse carefully documents the information that was provided to the client and that notification of the provider occurred. The client should be informed of the following.
  - Possible complications that could occur without treatment
  - Possibility of permanent physical or mental impairment or disability
  - Possibility of other complications that could lead to death
- The client is asked to sign an Against Medical Advice form.
- If the client refuses to sign the form, this is also documented by the nurse.

Advocacy

Advocacy refers to nurses' role in supporting clients by ensuring that they are properly informed, that their rights are respected, and that they are receiving the proper level of care.

- Advocacy is one of the most important roles of the nurse, especially when clients are unable to speak or act for themselves.
- As an advocate, the nurse ensures that the client has the information he needs to make decisions about health care.
- Nurses must act as advocates even when they disagree with clients' decisions.
- The complex health care system puts clients in a vulnerable position. Nurses are clients' voice when the system is not acting in their best interest.
- The nursing profession also has a responsibility to support and advocate for legislation that promotes public policies that protect clients as consumers and create a safe environment for their care.

NURSING ROLE IN ADVOCACY

- As advocates, nurses must ensure that clients are informed of their rights and have adequate information on which to base health care decisions.
- Nurses must be careful to assist clients with making health care decisions and not direct or control their decisions.
- Nurses mediate on the client's behalf when the actions of others are not in the client's best interest or changes need to be made in the plan of care.
- Situations in which nurses might need to advocate for clients or assist them to advocate for themselves include the following.
  - End-of-life decisions
  - Access to health care
  - Protection of client privacy
  - Informed consent
  - Substandard practice
- Nurses are accountable for their actions even if they are carrying out a provider's prescription. It is the nurse's responsibility to question a prescription if it could harm a client (incorrect medication dosage, potential adverse interaction with another prescribed medication, contraindication due to an allergy or medical history). Qs

ESSENTIAL COMPONENTS OF ADVOCACY

SKILLS
- Risk-taking
- Vision
- Self-confidence
- Articulate communication
- Assertiveness

VALUES
- Caring
- Autonomy
- Respect
- Empowerment

Informed consent

- Informed consent is a legal process by which a client has given written permission for a procedure or treatment to be performed. Consent is considered to be informed when the client has been provided with and understands the following.
  - Reason the treatment or procedure is needed
  - How the treatment or procedure will benefit the client
  - Risks involved if the client chooses to receive the treatment or procedure
  - Other options to treat the problem, including the option of not treating the problem
  - Risk involved if the client chooses no treatment
- The nurse's role in the informed consent process is to witness the client's signature on the informed consent form and to ensure that informed consent has been appropriately obtained.
- The nurse should seek the assistance of an interpreter if the client does not speak and understand the language used by the provider. Qpcc

INFORMED CONSENT GUIDELINES

Consent is required for all care given in a health care facility. For most aspects of nursing care, implied consent is adequate. The client provides implied consent when she complies with the instructions provided by the nurse. For example, the nurse is preparing to administer a TB skin test, and the client holds out her arm for the nurse.

- For an invasive procedure or surgery, the client is required to provide written consent.
- State laws regulate who is able to give informed consent. Laws vary regarding age limitations and emergencies. Nurses are responsible for knowing the laws in the state of practice.
- The nurse must verify that consent is informed and witness the client sign the consent form.

Signing an informed consent form

- The form for informed consent must be signed by a competent adult.
  - Emancipated minors (minors who are independent from their parents, such as a married minor) can provide informed consent for themselves.
- The person who signs the form must be capable of understanding the information provided by the health care professional who will be providing the service. The person must be able to fully communicate in return with the health care professional.
- When the person giving the informed consent is unable to communicate due to a language barrier or hearing impairment, a trained medical interpreter must be provided. Many health care agencies contract with professional interpreters who have additional skills in medical terminology to assist with providing information.

Individuals authorized to grant
consent for another person

- Parent of a minor
- Legal guardian
- Court-specified representative
- Client's health care surrogate (individual who has the client's durable power of attorney for health care/health care proxy)
- Spouse or closest available relative (state laws vary)

INFORMED CONSENT RESPONSIBILITIES

PROVIDER: Obtains informed consent. To do so, the provider must give the client the following

- Complete description of the treatment/procedure
- Description of the professionals who will be performing and participating in the treatment
- Description of the potential harm, pain, and/or discomfort that might occur
- Options for other treatments
- The right to refuse treatment
- Risk involved if the client chooses no treatment

CLIENT: Gives informed consent. To give informed consent, the client must do the following.

- Give it voluntarily (no coercion involved).
- Be competent and of legal age or be an emancipated minor. (If the client is unable to provide consent, an authorized person must give consent).
- Receive sufficient information to make a decision based on an informed understanding of what is expected.

NURSE

- Witnesses informed consent. The nurse is responsible for the following. **Qs**
  - Ensuring that the provider gave the client the necessary information
  - Ensuring that the client understood the information and is competent to give informed consent
  - Having the client sign the informed consent document
  - Notifying the provider if the client has more questions or does not understand any of the information provided. (The provider is then responsible for giving clarification.)
- The nurse documents the following.
  - Reinforcement of information originally given by the provider
  - That questions the client had were forwarded to the provider
  - Use of an interpreter

Advance directives

- The purpose of advance directives is to communicate a client's wishes regarding end-of-life care should the client become unable to do so.
- The PSDA requires that all clients admitted to a health care facility be asked if they have advance directives.
  - A client who does not have advance directives must be given written information that outlines her rights related to health care decisions and how to formulate advance directives. Qᴘᴄᴄ
  - A health care representative should be available to help with this process.

COMPONENTS OF ADVANCE DIRECTIVES

Two components of an advance directive are the living will and the durable power of attorney for health care.

Living will

- A living will is a legal document that expresses the client's wishes regarding medical treatment in the event the client becomes incapacitated and is facing end-of-life issues. Types of treatments that are often addressed in a living will are those that have the capacity to prolong life. Examples of treatments that are addressed are cardiopulmonary resuscitation, mechanical ventilation, and feeding by artificial means.
- Living wills are legal in all states. However, state statutes and individual health care facility policies can vary. Nurses need to be familiar with their state statute and facility policies.
- Most state laws include provisions that health care providers who follow the health care directive in a living will are protected from liability.

Durable power of attorney for health care

A durable power of attorney for health care/health care proxy is a legal document that designates a health care surrogate, who is an individual authorized to make health care decisions for a client who is unable.

- The person who serves in the role of health care surrogate to make decisions for the client should be very familiar with the client's wishes.
- Living wills can be difficult to interpret, especially in the face of unexpected circumstances. A durable power of attorney for health care, as an adjunct to a living will, can be a more effective way of ensuring that the client's decisions about health care are honored.

Provider's prescriptions

- Unless a do not resuscitate (DNR) or allow natural death (AND) prescription is written, the nurse should initiate CPR when a client has no pulse or respirations. The written prescription for a DNR or AND must be placed in the client's medical record. The provider consults the client and the family prior to administering a DNR or AND.
- Additional prescriptions by the provider are based on the client's individual needs and decisions and provide for comfort measures. The client's decision is respected in regard to the use of antibiotics, initiation of diagnostic tests, and provision of nutrition by artificial means.

NURSING ROLE IN ADVANCE DIRECTIVES

- Providing written information regarding advance directives
- Documenting the client's advance directives status
- Ensuring that advance directives are current and reflective of the client's current decisions
- Recognizing that the client's choice takes priority when there is a conflict between the client and family, or between the client and the provider
- Informing all members of the health care team of the client's advance directives Qᴘᴄᴄ

Advance Directive
Living Will/Power of Attorney for Health Care

On this _____ day of _____ , I, _____ , being of sound mind, willfull designate the following individual,_____ , as my agent to make all health care related decisions for me.

If, for any reason, should I revoke my agent's authority of if my agent is not willing, able, or available to make health care decisions for me, I designate as my first alternate, _____

MY AGENT shall have the authority to make health care decisions that will become effective if and when my primary physician determines that I am unable, either physically and/or mentally, to make my own decisions regarding my health care.

MY AGENT shall have the authority to make health care decisions in what he/she determines is my best interest and carry out any instructions that I mark as my own will to be done.

MY AGENT shall be in accordance with my following choice:

☐ Choice NOT to Prolong Life

I do not want to be resuscitated in the event I (1) have an incurable and irreversible condition that will result in my death within a short period of time, (2) become unconscious and have little or no chance of regaining consciousness, or (3) the risks of treatment would outweigh the expected benefits.

☐ Choice To Prolong Life

I want my life to be prolonged as long as possible within the scope and limits of accepted health care standards.

MY AGENT shall direct that treatment for alleviation of pain or discomfort should be provided at all times even if it directly affects the demise of my health or hastens my death.

MY AGENT shall donate my organs as specified below.

☐ I give all organs, tissues, or parts

☐ I give the following organs, tissues, or parts ONLY: _____

☐ My gift is for the following purposes (Place a mark in the box next to the desired purpose(s) for donation:

    ☐ Transplant

    ☐ Therapy

    ☐ Research

    ☐ Education

MY AGENT shall, upon my death, make health care decisions regarding authorization of any autopsy, making anatomical gifts, and the disposition of my remains.

This Power of Attorney will not be effective unless it is signed by me, my designated agent, my alternative agent and my primary physician.

Signature: _____ Date: _____

Signature: _____ Date: _____

Signature: _____ Date: _____

Physician Signature: _____ Date: _____

Confidentiality and information security

Clients have the right to privacy and confidentiality in relation to their health care information and medical recommendations.

- Nurses who disclose client information to an unauthorized person can be liable for invasion of privacy, defamation, or slander.
- The security and privacy rules of the Health Insurance Portability and Accountability Act (HIPAA) were enacted to protect the confidentiality of health care information and to give the client the right to control the release of information. Specific rights provided by the legislation include the following:
  - The rights of clients to obtain a copy of their medical record and to submit requests to amend erroneous or incomplete information
  - A requirement for health care and insurance providers to provide written information about how medical information is used and how it is shared with other entities (permission must be obtained before information is shared)
  - The rights of clients to privacy and confidentiality

NURSING ROLE IN CONFIDENTIALITY

It is essential for nurses to be aware of the rights of clients in regard to privacy and confidentiality. Facility policies and procedures are established in order to ensure compliance with HIPAA regulations. It is essential that nurses know and adhere to the policies and procedures. HIPAA regulations also provide for penalties in the event of noncompliance with the regulations. Qs

PRIVACY RULE

The Privacy Rule of HIPAA requires that nurses protect all written and verbal communication about clients.

COMPONENTS OF THE PRIVACY RULE

- Only health care team members directly responsible for the client's care are allowed access to the client's records. Nurses may not share information with other clients or staff not involved in the care of the client.
- Clients have a right to read and obtain a copy of their medical record, and agency policy should be followed when the client requests to read or have a copy of the record.
- No part of the client record can be copied except for authorized exchange of documents between health care institutions. For example:
  - Transfer from a hospital to an extended care facility
  - Exchange of documents between a general practitioner and a specialist during a consult

- Client medical records must be kept in a secure area to prevent inappropriate access to the information. Using public display boards to list client names and diagnoses is restricted.
- Electronic records should be password-protected, and care must be taken to prevent public viewing of the information. Health care workers should use only their own passwords to access information.
- Client information may not be disclosed to unauthorized individuals, including family members who request it and individuals who call on the phone.
  - Many hospitals use a code system in which information is only disclosed to individuals who can provide the code.
  - Nurses should ask any individual inquiring about a client's status for the code and disclose information only when an individual can give the code.
- Communication about a client should only take place in a private setting where it cannot be overheard by unauthorized individuals. The practice of "walking rounds," where other clients and visitors can hear what is being said, is no longer sanctioned. Taped rounds also are discouraged because nurses should not receive information about clients for whom they are not responsible. Change-of-shift reports can be done at the bedside as long as the client does not have a roommate and no unsolicited visitors are present. Qpcc

INFORMATION SECURITY

- Health information systems (HIS) are used to manage administrative functions and clinical functions. The clinical portion of the system is often referred to as the clinical information systems (CIS). The CIS may be used to coordinate essential aspects of client care. Qi
- In order to comply with HIPAA regulations, each health care facility has specific policies and procedures designed to monitor staff adherence, technical protocols, computer privacy, and data safety.

INFORMATION SECURITY PROTOCOLS

- Log off from the computer before leaving the workstation to ensure that others cannot view protected health information (PHI) on the monitor.
- Never share a user ID or password with anyone.
- Never leave a client's chart or other printed or written PHI where others can access it.
- Shred any printed or written client information used for reporting or client care after it is no longer needed.

USE OF SOCIAL MEDIA

- The use of social media by members of the nursing profession is common practice. The benefits to using social media are numerous. It provides a mechanism for nurses to access current information about health care and enhances communication among nurses, colleagues, and clients and families. It also provides an opportunity for nurses to express concerns and seek support from others. But nurses must be cautious about the risk of intentional or inadvertent breaches of confidentiality via social media.
- The right to privacy is a fundamental component of client care. Invasion of privacy as it relates to health care is the release of client health information to others without the client's consent. Confidentiality is the duty of the nurse to protect a client's private information.
- The inappropriate use of social media can result in a breach of client confidentiality. Depending on the circumstances, the consequences can include termination of employment by the employer, discipline by the board of nursing, charges of defamation or invasion of privacy, and in the most serious of circumstances, federal charges for violation of HIPAA.

PROTECTING YOURSELF AND OTHERS

- Become familiar with facility policies about the use of social media, and adhere to them.
- Avoid disclosing any client health information online. Be sure no one can overhear conversations about a client when speaking on the telephone.
- Do not take or share photos or videos of a client.
- Remember to maintain professional boundaries when interacting with clients online.
- Never post a belittling or offensive remark about a client, employer, or coworker.
- Report any violations of facility social media policies to the nurse manager.

Information technology

- Informatics is the use of computers to systematically resolve issues in nursing. The use of technology in healthcare is increasing and most forms of communication are in electronic format. Qu
- Examples of how a nurse can use the electronic format while providing client care include laptops for documentation and the use an of automated medication dispensing system to dispense medications.
- Databases on diseases and medications are available for the nurse to review. These databases can also be used as a teaching tool when nurses are educating clients.
- The nurse can review medications, diseases, procedures, and treatments using an electronic format.
- Computers can be beneficial for use with clients who have visual impairments.
- The Internet is a valuable tool for clients to review current medications and or health questions. This is especially true for clients who have chronic illnesses.
- Nurses should instruct clients to only review valid and credible websites by verifying the author, institution, credentials, and how current the article is. A disclaimer will be presented if information is not medical advice.
- Clients can access their electronic health record (EHR) which is part of e-health. E-health enables the client to make appointments online, review laboratory results, refill an electronic prescription, and review billing information. The goal of e-health is improved health care outcomes due to 24 hr access by the client and provider to the client's health care information.

Legal practice

In order to be safe practitioners, nurses must understand the legal aspects of the nursing profession. Qs

- Understanding the laws governing nursing practice allows nurses to protect client rights and reduce the risk of nursing liability.
- Nurses are accountable for practicing nursing in accordance with the various sources of law affecting nursing practice. It is important that nurses know and comply with these laws. By practicing nursing within the confines of the law, nurses are able to do the following.
  - Provide safe, competent care
  - Advocate for clients' rights
  - Provide care that is within the nurse's scope of practice
  - Discern the responsibilities of nursing in relation to the responsibilities of other members of the health care team
  - Provide care that is consistent with established standards of care.
  - Shield oneself from liability

SOURCES OF LAW

Federal regulations

Federal regulations have a great impact on nursing practice. Some of the federal laws affecting nursing practice include the following.
- HIPAA
- Americans with Disabilities Act (ADA)
- Mental Health Parity Act (MHPA)
- Patient Self-Determination Act
- Uniform Anatomical Gift Act
- National Organ Transplant Act

Criminal and civil laws

Criminal law is a subsection of public law and relates to the relationship of an individual with the government. Violations of criminal law can be categorized as either a **felony** (a serious crime, such as homicide) or **misdemeanor** (a less serious crime, such as petty theft). A nurse who falsifies a record to cover up a serious mistake can be found guilty of breaking a criminal law.

Civil laws protect the individual rights of people. One type of civil law that relates to the provision of nursing care is tort law. Torts can be classified as unintentional, quasi-intentional, or intentional.

Unintentional torts
- **Negligence:** Practice or misconduct that does not meet expected standards of care and places the client at risk for injury (a nurse fails to implement safety measures for a client who has been identified as at risk for falls).
- **Malpractice:** Professional negligence (a nurse administers a large dose of medication due to a calculation error. The client has a cardiac arrest and dies).

Quasi-intentional torts
- **Invasion of privacy:** Intrusion into a client's private affairs or a breach of confidentiality (a nurse releases the medical diagnosis of a client to a member of the press).
- **Defamation:** False communication or communication with careless disregard for the truth with the intent to injure an individual's reputation.
  - **Libel:** Defamation with the written word or photographs (a nurse documents in a client's health record that a provider is incompetent).
  - **Slander:** Defamation with the spoken word (a nurse tells a coworker that she believes a client has been unfaithful to the spouse).

Intentional torts
- **Assault:** The conduct of one person makes another person fearful and apprehensive (threatening to place a nasogastric tube in a client who is refusing to eat).
- **Battery:** Intentional and wrongful physical contact with a person that involves an injury or offensive contact (restraining a client and administering an injection against his wishes).
- **False imprisonment:** A person is confined or restrained against his will (using restraints on a competent client to prevent his leaving the health care facility).

State laws

- The core of nursing practice is regulated by state law.
- Each state has enacted statutes that define the parameters of nursing practice and give the authority to regulate the practice of nursing to its state board of nursing.
  - Boards of nursing have the authority to adopt rules and regulations that further regulate nursing practice. Although the practice of nursing is similar among states, it is critical that nurses know the laws and rules governing nursing in the state in which they practice.
  - The laws and rules governing nursing practice in a specific state can be accessed at the state board's Web site.
  - Boards of nursing have the authority to both issue and revoke a nursing license. Boards may revoke or suspend a nurse's license for a number of offenses, including practicing without a valid license, substance use disorders, conviction of a felony, professional negligence, and providing care beyond the scope of practice. Nurses should review the practice act in their states.
  - Boards also set standards for nursing programs and further delineate the scope of practice for registered nurses, licensed practical nurses, and advanced practice nurses.

Good Samaritan laws

- Good Samaritan laws, which vary from state to state, protect nurses who provide emergency assistance outside of the employment location. The nurse must provide a standard of care that is reasonable and prudent.
- State laws vary as to when an individual may begin practicing nursing. Some states allow graduates of nursing programs to practice under a limited license, whereas some states require licensure by passing the NCLEX® before working.

Licensure

- Until the year 2000, nurses were required to hold a current license in every state in which they practiced. This became problematic with the increase in the electronic practice of nursing. For example, a nurse in one state interprets the reading of a cardiac monitor and provides intervention for a client who is physically located in another state. Additionally, many nurses cross state lines to provide direct care. For example, a nurse who is located near a state border makes home visits on both sides of the state line.
- To address these issues, the mutual recognition model of nurse licensure (the Nurse Licensure Compact [NLC]) has been adopted by many states. This model allows nurses who reside in a NLC state to practice in another NLC state. Nurses must practice in accordance with the statues and rules of the state in which the care is provided. State boards may prohibit a nurse from practicing under the NLC if the license of the nurse has been restricted by a board of nursing.
- Nurses who do not reside in a NLC state must practice under the state-based practice model. In other words, if a nurse resides in a non-NLC state, the nurse must maintain a current license in every state in which she practices. Some states now require background checks with licensure renewal. It is illegal to practice nursing with an expired license.

MALPRACTICE (PROFESSIONAL NEGLIGENCE)

- Malpractice is the failure of a person with professional training to act in a reasonable and prudent manner. The terms "reasonable and prudent" are generally used to describe a person who has the average judgment, foresight, intelligence, and skill that would be expected of a person with similar training and experience. **(3.2)**
- Professional negligence issues that prompt most malpractice suits include failure to do the following.
  - Follow either professional or facility established standards of care
  - Use equipment in a responsible and knowledgeable manner
  - Communicate effectively and thoroughly with the client
  - Document care that was provided
- Nurses can avoid being liable for negligence by doing the following.
  - Following standards of care
  - Giving competent care
  - Communicating with other health team members
  - Developing a caring rapport with clients
  - Fully documenting assessments, interventions, and evaluations

---

3.2 Elements necessary to prove negligence

	EXAMPLE: CLIENT WHO IS A FALL RISK
1. Duty to provide care as defined by a standard Care that should be given or what a reasonably prudent nurse would do	The nurse should complete a fall risk assessment for all clients upon admission, per facility protocol.
2. Breach of duty by failure to meet standard Failure to give the standard of care that should have been given	The nurse does not perform a fall risk assessment during admission.
3. Foreseeability of harm Knowledge that failing to give the proper standard of care can cause harm to the client	The nurse should know that failure to take fall-risk precautions can endanger a client at risk for falls.
4. Breach of duty has potential to cause harm (combines elements 2 and 3) Failure to meet the standard had potential to cause harm: relationship must be provable	If a fall risk assessment is not performed, the client's risk for falls is not determined and the proper precautions are not put in place.
5. Harm occurs Occurrence of actual harm to the client	The client falls out of bed and breaks his hip.

STANDARDS OF CARE (PRACTICE)

- Nurses base practice on established standards of care or legal guidelines for care. These standards of care can be found in the following.
  - The nurse practice act of each state
    - These acts govern nursing practice, and legal guidelines for practice are established and enforced through a state board of nursing or other government agency.
    - Nurse practice acts vary from state to state, making it obligatory for the nurse to be informed about her state's nurse practice act as it defines the legal parameters of practice.
  - Published standards of nursing practice: These are developed by professional organizations such as the American Nurses Association, National Association of Practical Nurse Education and Services, Inc., and specialty organizations such as the American Association of Critical Care Nurses, Wound, Ostomy and Continence Nurses Society; and Oncology Nurses Society.
  - Accrediting bodies (e.g., The Joint Commission)
  - Originally mandated quality assurance programs, which have evolved into quality improvement
  - Sentinel event reporting: "An unexpected occurrence involving death or serious or psychological injury, or the risk thereof"
  - Failure Mode and Effects Analysis: Examines all potential failures in a design, including event sequencing risks, vulnerabilities, and improvement areas
  - National Patient Safety Goals: Augments core measures and promotes patient safety through patient identification, effective staff communication, safe medication use, infection prevention, safety risk identification, and preventing wrong-site surgery
  - Health care facility policies and procedures
    - Policies and procedures, maintained in the facility's policy and procedure manual, establish the standard of practice for employees of that institution.
    - These manuals provide detailed information about how the nurse should respond to or provide care in specific situations and while performing client care procedures.
    - Nurses who practice according to institutional policy are legally protected if that standard of care still results in an injury. For example, if a client files a complaint with the board of nursing or seeks legal counsel, the nurse who has followed the facility's policies will not usually be charged with misconduct.
    - It is very important that nurses are familiar with their institution's policies and procedures and provide client care in accordance with these policies. For example:
      - Assess and document findings postoperatively according to institutional policy.
      - Change IV tubing and flush saline locks according to institutional policy.
- Standards of care guide, define, and direct the level of care that should be given by practicing nurses. They also are used in malpractice lawsuits to determine if that level was maintained.
- Nurses should refuse to practice beyond the legal scope of practice and/or outside of their areas of competence regardless of reason (staffing shortage, lack of appropriate personnel).
- Nurses should use the formal chain of command to verbalize concerns related to assignment in light of current legal scope of practice, job description, and area of competence.

IMPAIRED COWORKERS

- Impaired health care providers pose a significant risk to client safety. Qs
- A nurse who suspects a coworker of using alcohol or other substances while working has a duty to report the coworker to appropriate management personnel as specified by institutional policy. At the time of the infraction, the report should be made to the immediate supervisor, such as the charge nurse, to ensure client safety.
- Health care facility policies should provide guidelines for handling employees who have a substance use disorder. Many facilities provide peer assistance programs that facilitate the health care provider's entry into a treatment program.
- Each state board of nursing has laws and regulations that govern the disposition of nurses who have been reported secondary to substance use. Depending on the individual case, the boards have the option to require the nurse to enter a treatment program, during which time the nurse's license can be retained, suspended, or revoked. If a nurse is allowed to maintain licensure, there usually are work restrictions put in place, such as working in noncritical care areas and being restricted from administering controlled medications.
- Health care providers who are found guilty of misappropriation of controlled substances also can be charged with a criminal offense consistent with the infraction.
- Behaviors can be difficult to detect if the impaired nurse is experienced at masking the substance use disorder.

BEHAVIORS CONSISTENT WITH A SUBSTANCE USE DISORDER

- Smell of alcohol on breath or frequent use of strong mouthwash or mints
- Impaired coordination, sleepiness, shakiness, and/or slurred speech
- Bloodshot eyes
- Mood swings and memory loss
- Neglect of personal appearance
- Excessive use of sick leave, tardiness, or absences after a weekend off, holiday, or payday
- Frequent requests to leave the unit for short periods of time or to leave the shift early
- Frequently "forgetting" to have another nurse witness wasting of a controlled substance
- Frequent involvement in incidences where a client assigned to the nurse reports not receiving pain medication or adequate pain relief (impaired nurse provides questionable explanations)
- Documenting administration of pain medication to a client who did not receive it or documenting a higher dosage than has been given by other nurses
- Preferring to work the night shift where supervision is less or on units where controlled substances are more frequently given

MANDATORY REPORTING

In certain situations, health care providers have a legal obligation to report their findings in accordance with state law.

ABUSE

- All 51 jurisdictions (50 states and the District of Colombia) have statutes requiring report of suspicion of child abuse. The statutes set out which occupations are mandatory reporters. In many states, nurses are mandatory reporters.
- A number of states also mandate that health care providers, including nurses, report suspected abuse of vulnerable persons, such as older or dependent adults.
- Nurses are mandated to report any suspicion of abuse following facility policy.

COMMUNICABLE DISEASES

- Nurses are also mandated to report to the proper agency (local health department, state health department) when a client is diagnosed with a communicable disease. Qs
- A complete list of reportable diseases and a description of the reporting system are available through the Centers for Disease Control and Prevention Web site, www.cdc.gov. Each state mandates which diseases must be reported in that state. There are more than 60 communicable diseases that must be reported to public health departments to allow officials to do the following.
  - Ensure appropriate medical treatment of diseases (tuberculosis).
  - Monitor for common-source outbreaks (foodborne: hepatitis A).
  - Plan and evaluate control and prevention plans (immunizations for preventable diseases).
  - Identify outbreaks and epidemics.
  - Determine public health priorities based on trends.
  - Educate the community on prevention and treatment of these diseases.

ORGAN DONATION

- Organ and tissue donation is regulated by federal and state laws. Health care facilities have policies and procedures to guide health care workers involved with organ donation.
- Donations may be stipulated in a will or designated on an official card.
- Federal law requires health care facilities to provide access to trained specialists who make the request to clients and/or family members and provide information regarding consent, organ and tissues that can be donated, and how burial or cremation will be affected by donation.
- Nurses are responsible for answering questions regarding the donation process and for providing emotional support to family members.

TRANSCRIBING MEDICAL PRESCRIPTIONS

- Nurses might need to receive new prescriptions for client care or medications by verbal or telephone prescription.
- When transcribing a prescription into a paper or electronic chart, nurses must do the following.
  - Be sure to include all necessary elements of a prescription: date and time prescription was written; new client care prescription or medication including dosage, frequency, route of administration; and signature of nurse transcribing the prescription as well as the provider who verbally gave the prescription.
  - Follow institutional policy with regard to the time frame within which the provider must sign the prescription (usually within 24 hr).
  - Use strategies to prevent errors when taking a medical prescription that is given verbally or over the phone by the provider.
    - Repeat back the prescription given, making sure to include the medication name (spell if necessary), dosage, time, and route. Qs
    - Question any prescription that seems contraindicated due to a previous or concurrent prescription or client condition.

Disruptive behavior

- Nurses experience incivility, lateral violence, and bullying at an alarming rate. The perpetrator can be a provider or a nursing colleague. Consequences of disruptive behavior include poor communication, which can negatively affect client safety and productivity, resulting in absenteeism, decreased job satisfaction, and staff turnover. Some nurses may choose to leave the profession due to these counterproductive behaviors.
- If disruptive behavior is allowed to continue, it is likely to escalate. Over time, it can be viewed as acceptable in that unit or department's culture.

TYPES OF DISRUPTIVE BEHAVIOR

- **Incivility** is defined as an action that is rude, intimidating, and insulting. It includes teasing, joking, dirty looks, and uninvited touching.
- **Lateral violence** is also known as horizontal abuse or horizontal hostility. It occurs between individuals who are at the same level within the organization. For example, a more experienced staff nurse can be abusive to a newly licensed nurse. Common behaviors include verbal abuse, undermining activities, sabotage, gossip, withholding information, and ostracism.
- **Bullying** behavior is persistent and relentless and is aimed at an individual who has limited ability to defend himself or herself. Bullying occurs when the perpetrator is at a higher level than the victim (for example, a nurse manager to a staff nurse). It is abuse of power that makes the recipient feel threatened, disgraced, and vulnerable. For example, a nurse manager can demonstrate favoritism for another nurse by making unfair assignments or refusing a promotion.
- **Cyberbullying** is a type of disruptive behavior using the Internet or other electronic means.

INTERVENTIONS TO DETER DISRUPTIVE BEHAVIORS

- Create an environment of mutual respect among staff.
- Model appropriate behavior.
- Increase staff awareness about disruptive behavior.
- Make staff aware that offensive online remarks about employers and coworkers are a form of bullying and are prohibited even if the nurse is off-duty and it is posted off-site from the facility.
- Avoid making excuses for disruptive behavior.
- Support zero tolerance for disruptive behavior.
- Establish mechanisms for open communication between staff nurses and nurse managers.
- Adopt policies that limit the risk of retaliation when disruptive behavior is reported.

Ethical practice

- **Ethics** has several definitions, but the foundation of ethics is based on an expected behavior of a certain group in relation to what is considered right and wrong.
- **Morals** are the values and beliefs held by a person that guide behavior and decision-making.
- **Ethical theory** analyzes varying philosophies, systems, ideas, and principles used to make judgments about what is right and wrong, good and bad. Two common types of ethical theory are utilitarianism and deontology.
  - Utilitarianism (teleological theory): Decision-making based on what provides the greatest good for the greatest number of individuals
  - Deontological theory: Decision-making based on obligations, duty, and what one considers to be right or wrong
- Unusual or complex ethical issues might need to be dealt with by a facility's ethics committee.

ETHICAL PRINCIPLES are standards of what is right or wrong with regard to important social values and norms. Ethical principles pertaining to the treatment of clients include the following. Qpcc

- **Autonomy:** The ability of the client to make personal decisions, even when those decisions might not be in the client's own best interest
- **Beneficence:** Care that is in the best interest of the client
- **Fidelity:** Keeping one's promise to the client about care that was offered
- **Justice:** Fair treatment in matters related to physical and psychosocial care and use of resources
- **Nonmaleficence:** The nurse's obligation to avoid causing harm to the client
- **Veracity:** The nurse's duty to tell the truth

3.3 The nurse's role in ethical decision-making

	EXAMPLES
An agent for the client facing an ethical decision	Caring for an adolescent client who is deciding whether to undergo an elective abortion even though her parents believe it is wrong
	Discussing options with parents who have to decide whether to consent to a blood transfusion for a child when their religion prohibits such treatment
A decision-maker in regard to nursing practice	Assigning staff nurses a higher client load than recommended because administration has cut the number of nurses per shift
	Witnessing a surgeon discuss only surgical options with a client without informing the client about more conservative measures available

ETHICAL DECISION-MAKING IN NURSING

Ethical dilemmas are problems for which more than one choice can be made, and the choice is influenced by the values and beliefs of the decision-makers. These are common in health care, and nurses must be prepared to apply ethical theory and decision-making.

- A problem is an ethical dilemma if:
  - It cannot be solved solely by a review of scientific data.
  - It involves a conflict between two moral imperatives.
  - The answer will have profound effect on the situation/client.
- Nurses have a responsibility to be advocates, and to identify and report ethical situations.
  - Doing so through the chain of command offers some protection against retribution.
  - Some state nurse associations offer protection for nurses who report substandard or unethical practice.
- Ethical decision-making is the process by which a decision is made about an ethical issue. Frequently, this requires a balance between science and morality. There are several steps in ethical decision-making:
  - Identify whether the issue is an ethical dilemma.
  - State the ethical dilemma, including all surrounding issues and individuals involved.
  - List and analyze all possible options for resolving the dilemma, and review implications of each option.
  - Select the option that is in concert with the ethical principle applicable to this situation, the decision maker's values and beliefs, and the profession's values set forth for client care. Justify why that one option was selected.
  - Apply this decision to the dilemma and evaluate the outcomes.

- The American Nurses Association Code of Ethics for Nurses (2001) and the International Council of Nurses' Code of Ethics for Nurses (2006) are commonly used by professional nurses. The Code of Ethics for Licensed Practical/Vocational Nurses issued by the National Association for Practical Nurse Education and Services also serves as a set of standards for Nursing Practice. Codes of ethics are available at the organizations' websites.
- The Uniform Determination of Death Act (UDDA) can be used to assist with end-of-life and organ donor issues.
  - The UDDA provides two formal definitions of death that were developed by the National Conference of Commissioners on Uniform State Laws. Death is determined by one of two criteria.
    - Irreversible cessation of circulatory and respiratory functions
    - Irreversible cessation of all functions of the entire brain, including the brain stem
  - A determination of death must be made in accordance with accepted medical standards.

PRACTICE Active Learning Scenario

A nurse is preparing to serve on a committee that will review the policy on disruptive behavior. Use the ATI Active Learning Template: Basic Concept to complete this item.

RELATED CONTENT: Describe another term used for lateral violence.

NURSING INTERVENTIONS: Describe at least four interventions to deter disruptive behavior.

Application Exercises

1. A nurse manager is observing the actions of a nurse she is supervising. Which of the following actions by the nurse requires the nurse manager to intervene? (Select all that apply.)

    A. Reviewing the health care record of a client assigned to another nurse

    B. Making a copy of a client's most current laboratory results for the provider during rounds

    C. Providing information about a client's condition to hospital clergy

    D. Discussing a client's condition over the phone with an individual who has provided the client's information code

    E. Participating in walking rounds that involve the exchange of client-related information outside clients' rooms

2. A nurse is caring for a client who is scheduled for surgery. The client hands the nurse information about advance directives and states, "Here, I don't need this. I am too young to worry about life-sustaining measures and what I want done for me." Which of the following actions should the nurse take?

    A. Return the papers to the admitting department with a note stating that the client does not wish to address the issue at this time.

    B. Explain to the client that you never know what can happen during surgery and that he should fill the papers out just in case.

    C. Contact a client representative to talk with the client and offer additional information about the purpose of advance directives.

    D. Inform the client that surgery cannot be conducted unless he completes the advance directives forms.

3. A nurse witnesses an assistive personnel (AP) under her supervision reprimanding a client for not using the urinal properly. The AP threatens to put a diaper on the client if he does not use the urinal more carefully next time. Which of the following torts is the AP committing?

    A. Assault

    B. Battery

    C. False imprisonment

    D. Invasion of privacy

4. A nurse is serving as a preceptor to a newly licensed nurse and is explaining the role of the nurse as advocate. Which of the following situations illustrates the advocacy role? (Select all that apply.)

    A. Verifying that a client understands what is done during a cardiac catheterization

    B. Discussing treatment options for a terminal diagnosis

    C. Informing members of the health care team that a client has do-not-resuscitate status

    D. Reporting that a health team member on the previous shift did not provide care as prescribed

    E. Assisting a client to make a decision about his care based on the nurse's recommendations

5. A nurse manager is providing information to the nurses on the unit about ensuring client rights. Which of the following regulations outlines the rights of individuals in health care settings?

    A. American Nurses Association Code of Ethics

    B. HIPAA

    C. Patient Self-Determination Act

    D. Patient Care Partnership

6. A newly licensed nurse is preparing to insert an IV catheter in a client. Which of the following sources should the nurse use to review the procedure and the standard at which it should be performed?

    A. Website

    B. Institutional policy and procedure manual

    C. More experienced nurse

    D. State nurse practice act

7. A nurse is reviewing a client's health care record and discovers that the client's do-not-resuscitate (DNR) prescription has expired. The client's condition is not stable. Which of the following actions should the nurse take?

    A. Assume that the client does not want to be resuscitated, and take no action if she experiences cardiac arrest.

    B. Write a note on the front of the provider prescription sheet asking that the DNR be represcribed.

    C. Anticipate that CPR will be instituted if the client goes into cardiopulmonary arrest.

    D. Call the provider to determine whether the prescription should be immediately reinstated.

8. A nurse is caring for a toddler who is being treated in the emergency department following a head contusion from a fall. History reveals the toddler lives at home with only her mother. The provider's discharge instructions include waking the child every hour to assess for indications of a possible head injury. In which of the following situations should the nurse intervene and attempt to prevent discharge?

    A. The mother states she does not have insurance or money for a follow-up visit.

    B. The child states her head hurts and she wants to go home.

    C. The nurse smells alcohol on the mother's breath.

    D. The mother verbalizes fear about taking the child home and requests she be kept overnight.

Application Exercises Key

1. A. **CORRECT:** To maintain confidentiality, client information is disseminated on a need-to-know basis only. A nurse who is not assigned to care for a client should not access the client's information.

    B. **CORRECT:** Paper copies of confidential information create a risk for breach of confidentiality.

    C. **CORRECT:** Information about a client's condition is disseminated on a need-to-know basis. It is inappropriate to share this information with the hospital clergy.

    D. The nurse can share information with an individual who has been provided the information code.

    E. **CORRECT:** Sharing information in the hallway where it can be overheard by others can result in a breach of confidentiality.

    Ⓝ *NCLEX® Connection: Management of Care, Assignment, Delegation and Supervision*

2. A. The nurse should advocate for the client by ensuring that the client understands the purpose of advance directives.

    B. This response is nontherapeutic and can cause the client to be anxious about the surgery.

    C. **CORRECT:** The nurse should advocate for the client by ensuring that the client understands the purpose of advance directives. Seeking the assistance of a client representative to provide information to the client is an appropriate action.

    D. This statement is untrue and is a barrier to therapeutic communication.

    Ⓝ *NCLEX® Connection: Management of Care, Advance Directives/Self-Determine/Life Planning*

3. A. **CORRECT:** Assault is conduct that makes a person fear he or she will be harmed.

    B. Battery is physical contact without a person's consent.

    C. False imprisonment is restraining a person against his or her will. It includes the use of physical or chemical restraints, and refusing to allow a client to leave a facility

    D. Invasion of privacy is the unauthorized release of a client's private information.

    Ⓝ *NCLEX® Connection: Management of Care, Concepts of Management*

4. A. **CORRECT:** Ensuring that the client has given informed consent illustrates nurse advocacy.

    B. Discussing treatment options is not within the scope of practice of the nurse.

    C. **CORRECT:** Ensuring that the client's care is consistent with his DNR status illustrates nurse advocacy.

    D. **CORRECT:** Ensuring that all clients receive proper care illustrates nurse advocacy.

    E. Assisting a client to make decisions about his care based on nurse recommendations is inappropriate. The nurse should support the client in making his own decisions.

    Ⓝ *NCLEX® Connection: Management of Care, Client Rights*

5. A. The American Nurses Association Code of Ethics provides nurses with a set of standards for nursing practice.

    B. The Privacy Rule of HIPAA ensures client privacy and confidentiality.

    C. The Patient Self-Determination Act is federal legislation that requires that all clients admitted to a health care facility be asked whether they have advance directives.

    D. **CORRECT:** The Patient Care Partnership is a document that addresses clients' rights when receiving care.

    Ⓝ *NCLEX® Connection: Management of Care, Information Technology*

6. A. A website might not provide information that is consistent with institutional policy.

    B. **CORRECT:** The institutional policy and procedure manual will provide instructions on how to perform the procedure that is consistent with established standards. This is the resource the nurse should use.

    C. A more experienced nurse on the unit might not perform the procedure according to the policy and procedure manual.

    D. The nurse practice act identifies scope of practice and other aspects of the law, but it does not set standards for performance of a procedure.

    Ⓝ *NCLEX® Connection: Management of Care, Advance Directives/Self-Determine/Life Planning*

7. A. Without a current DNR prescription, the nurse must initiate emergency resuscitation, which most likely is not consistent with the client's wishes.

    B. Without a current DNR prescription, the nurse must initiate emergency resuscitation, which most likely is not consistent with the client's wishes. Writing a note on the prescription sheet likely will result in a delay in resolving the problem.

    C. Without a current DNR prescription, the nurse must initiate emergency resuscitation, which most likely is not consistent with the client's wishes.

    D. **CORRECT:** The nurse should immediately call the provider to determine whether the prescription should be reinstated. This is the action to take to be sure that the client's wishes are carried out.

    Ⓝ *NCLEX® Connection: Management of Care, Advocacy*

8. A. Lack of insurance does not warrant a delay in discharge, but it can indicate the need for referral for social services to assist with client needs.

    B. The toddler's report of pain is an expected finding.

    C. **CORRECT:** It would be unsafe to discharge a toddler who requires hourly monitoring with a mother who might be chemically impaired.

    D. Fear verbalized by the mother does not warrant denial in discharge. The nurse should allay the mother's fears by educating her about how to monitor the child and provide phone numbers for the mother to use.

    Ⓝ *NCLEX® Connection: Management of Care, Ethical Practice*

PRACTICE Answer

Using ATI Active Learning Template: Basic Concept

RELATED CONTENT: Lateral violence is also known as horizontal abuse or horizontal hostility.

NURSING INTERVENTIONS

- Create an environment of mutual respect among staff.
- Model appropriate behavior.
- Increase staff awareness about disruptive behavior.
- Make staff aware that offensive online remarks about employers and coworkers are a form of bullying and is prohibited even if the nurse is off-duty and it is posted off-site of the facility.
- Avoid making excuses for disruptive behavior.
- Support zero tolerance for disruptive behavior.
- Establish mechanisms for open communication between staff nurses and nurse managers.
- Adopt policies that limit the risk of retaliation when disruptive behavior is reported.

Ⓝ *NCLEX® Connection: Management of Care, Concepts of Management*

When reviewing the following chapter, keep in mind the relevant topics and tasks of the NCLEX outline, in particular:

Client Needs: Safety and Infection Control

CHANGE TO ACCIDENT/ERROR/INJURY PREVENTION: Determine client/staff member knowledge of safety procedures.

HANDLING HAZARDOUS AND INFECTIOUS MATERIALS: Follow procedures for handling biohazardous materials.

HOME SAFETY: Evaluate client care environment for fire/environmental hazards.

SAFE USE OF EQUIPMENT: Facilitate appropriate and safe use of equipment.

STANDARD PRECAUTIONS/TRANSMISSION-BASED PRECAUTIONS/SURGICAL ASEPSIS: Educate client and staff regarding infection control measures.

Maintaining a Safe Environment

Maintaining a safe environment refers to the precautions and considerations required to ensure that physical environments are safe for clients and staff. Qs

Knowing how to maintain client safety has been identified by the Institute of Medicine as a competency that graduates of nursing programs must possess.

Quality and Safety Education for Nurses (QSEN) faculty propose that nursing education focus not only on the knowledge needed to provide safe care but also on the skills and attitudes that accompany this competency.

To maintain a safe environment, nurses must have knowledge, skills, and attitudes about QSEN competencies, handling infectious and hazardous materials, safe use of equipment, accident and injury prevention, home safety, and ergonomic principles.

QSEN competencies in nursing programs

Concern about the quality and safety of health care in the U.S. has prompted numerous reports and initiatives designed to address this issue. Data from the Joint Commission identify poor communication as a key factor in the majority of sentinel events. The Institute of Medicine (IOM) report *To Err is Human: Building a Safer Health System* (1999) spoke to the frequency of unnecessary deaths and preventable medical errors, and identified system failure as a major factor. Subsequent publications pointed to the need to redesign the provision of client care and improve education of students in health care programs.

The QSEN project identified specific competencies to include in each prelicensure nursing curriculum. These six competencies are now integral components of the curriculum of many nursing programs in the U.S.

Qpcc **PATIENT-CENTERED CARE:** The provision of caring and compassionate, culturally sensitive care that addresses clients' physiological, psychological, sociological, spiritual, and cultural needs, preferences, and values.

Qtc **TEAMWORK AND COLLABORATION:** The delivery of client care in partnership with multidisciplinary members of the health care team to achieve continuity of care and positive client outcomes.

Qebp **EVIDENCE-BASED PRACTICE:** The use of current knowledge from research and other credible sources on which to base clinical judgment and client care.

Qqi **QUALITY IMPROVEMENT:** Care-related and organizational processes that involve the development and implementation of a plan to improve health care services and better meet clients' needs.

Qs **SAFETY:** The minimization of risk factors that could cause injury or harm while promoting quality care and maintaining a secure environment for clients, self, and others.

Qi **INFORMATICS:** The use of information technology as a communication and information-gathering tool that supports clinical decision-making and scientifically-based nursing practice.

Handling infectious and hazardous materials

- Handling infectious and hazardous materials refers to infection control procedures and to precautions for handling toxic, radioactive, or other hazardous materials. Qs
- Safety measures are taken to protect the client, nurse, and other personnel and individuals from harmful materials and organisms.
- Four levels of precautions (standard, airborne, droplet, contact) are recommended for individuals coming in contact with clients carrying infectious organisms. Precautions consistent with the infectious organism should be followed as indicated.
- A manual containing safety data sheets (SDSs) should be available in every workplace and provide safety information, such as level of toxicity, handling and storage guidelines, and first aid and containment measures to take in case of accidental release of toxic, radioactive, or other dangerous materials. This manual should be available to all employees and can be housed in a location such as the emergency department of a hospital.

INFECTION CONTROL

Infection control is extremely important to prevent cross-contamination of communicable organisms and health care-associated infections.

- Staff education on infection prevention and control is a responsibility of the nurse.
- Facility policies and procedures should serve as a resource for proper implementation of infection prevention and control.
- Clients suspected of or known to have a communicable disease should be placed in the appropriate form of isolation.
- The nurse should ensure that appropriate equipment is available and that isolation procedures are properly carried out by all health care team members.
- Use of standard precautions by all members of the health care team should be enforced. Employees who are allergic to latex should have non-latex gloves (e.g., nitrile or vinyl) made available to them. A latex-free environment is provided for clients who have a latex allergy. Many facilities avoid the use of latex products unless there is no other alternative.
- Hand hygiene facilities, as well as hand sanitizer, must be readily accessible to employees in client care areas.
- Sturdy, moisture-resistant bags (usually red) should be used for soiled items, and the bags should be tied securely with a knot at the top. Double-bagging is not cost-effective and is unnecessary unless the outside of a bag becomes contaminated.

- Retractable needles or needles with capping mechanisms, needleless syringes, and IV tubing with needleless connections should be available for use to prevent accidental needlesticks. Education on how to safely use these devices for administration of intermittent infusions will prevent misuse during client care and staff injuries from improper manipulation.
- Sharps containers should be readily available in client care areas, and any needlestick involving an employee should be reported in accordance with facility policy and state law. An incident or occurrence report should also be filed. Most policies include testing of the client and nurse for blood-borne illnesses such as hepatitis and human immunodeficiency virus (HIV).

HAZARDOUS MATERIALS

- Nurses and other members of the health care team are at risk for exposure to hazardous materials.
- Employees have the right to refuse to work in hazardous working conditions if there is a clear threat to their health.
- Health care team members should follow occupational safety and health guidelines as set by the Occupational Safety and Health Administration (OSHA).
  - Provide each employee a work environment that is free from recognized hazards that can cause or are likely to cause death or serious physical harm.
  - Make protective gear accessible to employees working under hazardous conditions or with hazardous materials (antineoplastic medications, sterilization chemicals).
  - Provide measurement devices and keeping records that document an employee's level of exposure over time to hazardous materials, such as radiation from x-rays.
  - Provide education and recertification opportunities to each employee regarding these rules and regulations, such as handling of hazardous materials.
  - Maintain SDSs and ensure their availability to all employees.
  - Designate an institutional hazardous materials (HAZMAT) response team that responds to hazardous events.

HANDLING INFECTIOUS AND HAZARDOUS MATERIALS

- Members of the health care team must clean and maintain equipment that is shared by clients on a unit (blood pressure cuffs, thermometers, pulse oximeters).
- Keep designated equipment in the rooms of clients who are on contact precautions.
- Use standard precautions at all times.
- Employ proper hand hygiene techniques.
- Use needlestick precautions when handling needles and sharps.
- Maintain knowledge of rules and regulations and proper procedures for handling infectious/hazardous materials (use of red biohazard bag for disposal of contaminated materials, use of puncture-proof containers for sharps).

Safe use of equipment

- Safe use of equipment refers to appropriate operation of health care-related equipment by trained staff. Equipment-related injuries can occur as a result of malfunction, disrepair, or mishandling of mechanical equipment. Qs
- Nurses must ensure that they have the competence necessary to use equipment for tasks that fall within their scope of practice. Nurses should use equipment only after receiving sufficient instruction.
- Equipment should be regularly inspected by the engineering or maintenance department and by the user prior to use. Faulty equipment (frayed cords, disrepair) can start a fire or cause an electrical shock and should be removed from use and reported immediately per agency policy.

Nurses' responsibilities related to equipment safety

- Learning how to use and maintaining competency in the use of equipment
- Checking that equipment is accurately set and functioning properly (oxygen, nasogastric suction) at the beginning and during each shift
- Ensuring that electrical equipment is grounded (three-pronged plug and grounded outlet) to decrease the risk for electrical shock
- Ensuring that outlet covers are used in environments with individuals at risk for sticking items into them
- Unplugging equipment using the plug, not the cord, to prevent bending the plug prongs, which increases the risk for electrical shock
- Ensuring that life-support equipment is plugged into outlets designated to be powered by a backup generator during power outages
- Disconnecting all electrical equipment prior to cleaning
- Ensuring that all pumps (general and PCA) have free-flow protection to prevent an overdose of fluids or medications
- Ensuring that outlets are not overcrowded and that extension cords are used only when absolutely necessary (if they must be used in an open area, tape the cords to the floor)
- Using all equipment only as it is intended
- Immediately removing nonworking equipment from the client care area and sending it to the proper department for repair or disposal

Accident and injury prevention

- Preventing injury is a major nursing responsibility. Many factors affect a client's ability to protect himself. Qs
  - Age (pediatric and older adult clients are at greater risk)
  - Mobility
  - Cognitive and sensory awareness
  - Emotional state
  - Lifestyle and safety awareness
- All health care workers must be aware of the following.
  - How to assess for and recognize clients at risk for safety issues
  - Procedural safety guidelines
  - Protocols for responding to dangerous situations
  - Security plans
  - Identification and documentation of incidents and responses per health care agency policy

FALLS

Prevention of client falls is a major nursing priority. Nurses should assess all clients admitted to health care facilities for risk factors related to falls. Based on assessment findings, the nurse should implement preventative measures.

- Older adult clients can be at an increased risk for falls due to decreased strength, impaired mobility and balance, endurance limitations, and decreased sensory perception. Ⓖ
- Other risk factors include decreased visual acuity, generalized weakness, orthopedic problems (diabetic neuropathy), urinary frequency, gait and balance problems (Parkinson's disease, osteoporosis, arthritis), and cognitive dysfunction. Adverse effects of medications (orthostatic hypotension, drowsiness) also can increase the risk for falls.
- Clients are at greater risk for falls when multiple risk factors are present.

PREVENTION OF FALLS Qs

- Complete a fall risk assessment on the client upon admission and at regular intervals.
- The plan for each client is individualized based on the fall risk assessment findings.
- For example, if the client has orthostatic hypotension, instruct the client to avoid getting up too quickly, to sit on the side of the bed for a few seconds prior to standing, and to stand at the side of the bed for a few seconds prior to walking.

GENERAL MEASURES TO PREVENT FALLS

- Be sure the client knows how to use the call light, that it is in reach, and encourage its use.
- Respond to call lights in a timely manner.
- Orient the client to the setting (grab bars, call light), and ensure that the client understands how to use all assistive devices and can locate necessary items.
- Place clients at risk for falls near the nursing station.
- Ensure that bedside tables and overbed tables and frequently used items (telephone, water, tissues, call light) are within the client's reach.
- Maintain the bed in low position.
- Keep bed rails up and the bed in the low position for clients who are sedated, unconscious, or otherwise compromised.
- Avoid using full side bed rails for clients who get out of bed or attempt to get out of bed without assistance.
- Provide the client with nonskid footwear.
- Keep the floor free from clutter with a clear path to the bathroom (no scatter rugs, cords, furniture).
- Ensure adequate lighting
- Keep assistive devices (glasses, walkers, transfer devices) nearby after validation of safe use by the client and family.
- Educate the client and family/caregivers on identified risks and the plan of care.
- Lock wheels on beds, wheelchairs, and carts to prevent the device from rolling during transfers or stops.
- Use chair or bed sensors to alert staff of independent ambulation for clients at risk for getting up unattended.
- Report and document all incidents per agency policy. This provides valuable information that can be helpful in preventing similar incidents.
- To evaluate incidence of client falls, a formula based on 1,000 client days can be used. Using this formula, a facility can compare its fall rates to other facilities.

> (Number of client falls ÷ number of client days)
> × 1,000 = fall rate per 1,000 client days

SEIZURES

A seizure is a sudden surge of electrical activity in the brain. Seizures can occur at any time during a person's life and can be due to epilepsy, fever, or a variety of medical conditions. Partial seizures are due to electrical surges in one part of the brain, and generalized seizures involve the entire brain.

SEIZURE PRECAUTIONS

Seizure precautions (measures to protect the client from injury should a seizure occur) are taken for clients who have a history of seizures that involve the entire body or result in unconsciousness. Qs

- Ensure that rescue equipment, including oxygen, an oral airway, and suction equipment, is at the bedside. A saline lock can be placed for intravenous access if the client is at high risk for experiencing a generalized seizure.
- Inspect the client's environment for items that can cause injury in the event of a seizure, and remove items that are not necessary for current treatment.
- Assign the client to a room close to the nurses' station
- Assist the client who is at risk for a seizure with ambulation and transfers to reduce the risk of injury.
- Advise all caregivers and family not to put anything in the client's mouth in the event of a seizure.
- Advise all caregivers and family not to restrain the client in the event of a seizure. Instead, ensure safety by lowering the client to the floor if he is not in bed, protecting his head, removing nearby furniture, providing privacy, putting him on his side with his head slightly flexed forward if possible, and loosening clothing to prevent injury and promote dignity.
- In the event of a seizure, stay with the client, protect the client from injury, and call for help.
- Note the duration of the seizure and the sequence and type of movement.
- After a seizure, explain what happened to the client, and provide comfort, understanding, and a quiet environment for recovery.
- Document the seizure in the client's record along with any precipitating behaviors and a description of the event (movements, any injuries, length of seizure, aura, postictal state), and report it to the provider.

SECLUSION AND RESTRAINTS

Seclusion and restraints are used to prevent clients from injuring themselves or others.

- Seclusion is the placement of a client in a room that is private, isolated, and safe. Seclusion is used for clients who are at risk for injuring themselves or others.
- Physical restraint involves the application of a device that limits the client's movement. A restraint can limit the movement of the entire body or a body part.
- Chemical restraints are medications used to control the client's disruptive behavior.

RISKS ASSOCIATED WITH RESTRAINTS Qs

- Deaths by asphyxiation and strangulation have occurred with restraints.
- The client can also experience complications related to immobility, such as pressure ulcers, urinary and fecal incontinence, and pneumonia.

LEGAL CONSIDERATIONS

- Nurses should understand agency polices as well as federal and state laws that govern the use of restraints and seclusion.
- False imprisonment means the confinement of person without his consent. Improper use of restraints can subject the nurse to charges of false imprisonment.

GUIDELINES

- In general, seclusion and restraints should be prescribed for the shortest duration necessary and only if less restrictive measures have proved insufficient. They are for the physical protection of the client, or the protection of other clients or staff.
- Use of restraints is a difficult adjustment for the client and family. The client loses his freedom and can be embarrassed and experience low self-esteem and depression. The nurse can allay some of the concerns by explaining the purpose of the restraint and that the restraint is only temporary.
- Seclusion and/or restraints must never be used for
  - Convenience of the staff.
  - Punishment for the client.
  - Clients who are extremely physically or mentally unstable.
  - Clients who cannot tolerate the decreased stimulation of a seclusion room.
- PRN prescriptions for restraints are not permitted.

- Restraints should
  - Never interfere with treatment.
  - Restrict movement as little as is necessary to ensure safety.
  - Fit properly.
  - Be easily changed to decrease the chance of injury and to provide for the greatest level of dignity.
- When all other less restrictive means have been tried to prevent a client from harming self or others, the following must occur for seclusion or restraints to be used.
  - The treatment must be prescribed by the provider based on a face-to-face assessment of the client. In an emergency situation in which there is immediate risk to the client or others, the nurse can place a client in restraints. The nurse must obtain a prescription from the provider as soon as possible in accordance with agency policy (usually within 1 hr).
  - The prescription must specify the reason for the restraint, the type of restraint, the location of the restraint, how long the restraint can be used, and the type of behaviors demonstrated by the client that warrant use of the restraint.
  - The prescription allows for only 4 hr of restraints for an adult, 2 hr for clients age 9 to 17, and 1 hr for clients younger than 9 years of age. Providers may renew these prescriptions with a maximum of 24 consecutive hours.

NURSING RESPONSIBILITIES

Obtain a prescription from the provider for the restraint. If the client is at risk for harming self or others and a restraint is applied prior to consulting the provider, ensure that notification of the provider occurs in accordance with facility protocol.

- Conduct neurosensory checks every 2 hr or according to facility policy to include:
  - Circulation
  - Sensation
  - Mobility
- Offer food and fluids.
- Provide with means for hygiene and elimination.
- Monitor vital signs.
- Provide range of motion of extremities.
- Follow agency polices regarding restraints, including the need for signed consent from the client or guardian.
- Review the manufacturer's instructions for correct application.
- Remove or replace restraints frequently.
- Pad bony prominences.
- Use a quick-release knot to tie the restraint to the bed frame.
- Ensure that the restraint is loose enough for range of motion and has enough room to fit two fingers between the device and the client.
- Regularly assess the need for continued use of restraints.
- Never leave the client unattended without the restraint.

DOCUMENTATION

- Behavior or precipitating events that make the restraint necessary
- Attempts to use alternatives to restraints and the client's response
- Level of consciousness
- Type of restraint used and location
- Education/explanations to the client and family
- Exact time of application and removal
- Client behavior while restrained
- Type and frequency of care (range of motion, neurosensory checks, removal, integumentary checks)
- The client's response when the restraint is removed
- Medication administration

FIRE SAFETY

Fires in health care facilities are usually due to problems related to electrical or anesthetic equipment. Unauthorized smoking can also be the cause of a fire.

All staff must:
- Know the location of exits, alarms, fire extinguishers, and oxygen turnoff valves.
- Make sure equipment does not block fire doors.
- Know the evacuation plan for the unit and the facility.

Fire response follows the RACE sequence

R: Rescue and protect clients in close proximity to the fire by moving them to a safer location. Clients who are ambulatory may walk independently to a safe location.

A: Alarm: Activate the facility's alarm system and then report the fire's details and location.

C: Confine the fire by closing doors and windows and turning off any sources of oxygen and any electrical devices. Ventilate clients who are on life support with a bag-valve mask.

E: Extinguish the fire if possible using the appropriate fire extinguisher.

FIRE EXTINGUISHERS

To use a fire extinguisher, use the PASS sequence.

P: Pull the pin.

A: Aim at the base of the fire.

S: Squeeze the handle.

S: Sweep the extinguisher from side to side, covering the area of the fire.

Classes of fire extinguishers

Class A is for combustibles such as paper, wood, upholstery, rags, and other types of trash fires.

Class B is for flammable liquids and gas fires.

Class C is for electrical fires.

Home safety

In addition to taking measures to prevent injury to clients in a health care setting, nurses play a pivotal role in promoting safety in the client's home and community. Nurses often collaborate with the client, family, and members of the interprofessional team (social workers, occupational therapists, physical therapists) to promote client safety. Qs

Many factors contribute to the client's risk for injury.
- Age and developmental status
- Mobility and balance
- Knowledge about safety hazards
- Sensory and cognitive awareness
- Communication skills
- Home and work environment
- Community
- Medical and pharmacological status

To initiate a plan of care, the nurse must identify risk factors using a risk assessment tool and complete a nursing history, physical examination, and home hazard appraisal.

SAFETY RISKS BASED ON AGE AND DEVELOPMENTAL STATUS

- The age and developmental status of the client create specific safety risks. Qpcc
- Infants and toddlers are at risk for injury due to a tendency to put objects in their mouth and from hazards encountered while exploring their environment.
- Preschool- and school-age children often face injury from limited or underdeveloped motor coordination.
- Adolescents' risks for injury can stem from increased desire to make independent decisions, and relying on peers for guidance rather than family.
- Some of the accident prevention measures for specific age groups are found below.

INFANTS AND TODDLERS

Aspiration
- Keep all small objects out of reach.
- Check toys and objects for loose or small parts and sharp edges.
- Follow manufacturer recommendations for age appropriateness of toys.
- Do not feed the infant hard candy, peanuts, popcorn, or whole or sliced pieces of hot dog.
- Cut or break food that is age-appropriate into small bite-size pieces.
- Do not place the infant in the supine position while feeding or prop the infant's bottle.
- A pacifier (if used) should be constructed of one piece and never placed on string or ribbon around the neck.

Suffocation

- Teach "back to sleep" mnemonic and always place infants on back to rest.
- Keep plastic bags out of reach.
- Make sure crib mattress fits snugly and that crib slats are no more than 2 3/8 inches apart.
- Teach parents that it is recommended for infants to sleep in a crib or bassinet. Co-sleeping in bed with parents increases the risk for injury.
- Never leave an infant or toddler unattended in the bathtub.
- Do not place anything in crib with infant.
- Remove crib toys, such as mobiles, from over the bed as soon as the infant begins to push up.
- Keep latex balloons away from infants and toddlers.
- Fence swimming pools and use a locked gate.
- Begin swimming lessons when the child's developmental status allows for protective responses, such as closing her mouth under water.
- Teach caregivers CPR and Heimlich maneuver.
- Keep toilet lids down and bathroom doors closed.

Poisoning

- Keep houseplants and cleaning agents out of reach.
- Inspect and remove sources of lead, such as paint chips, and provide parents with information about prevention of lead poisoning.
- Place poisons, paint, and gasoline in locked cabinet.
- Keep medications in child-proof containers and locked up.
- Properly dispose of medications that are no longer used or are out of date.

Falls

- Keep crib and playpen rails up.
- Never leave the infant unattended on a changing table or other high surface.
- Use gates on stairs, and ensure windows have screens.
- Restrain according to manufacturer's recommendations and supervise when in high chair, swing, stroller, etc. Discontinue use when the infant or toddler outgrows size limits.
- Place in a low bed when toddler starts to climb.

Motor vehicle injury

- Place infants and toddlers in a rear-facing car seat until 2 years of age or until they exceed the height and weight limit of the car seat. They can then sit in a forward-facing car seat.
- Use a car seat with a five-point harness for infants and children.
- All car seats should be federally approved and be placed in the back seat.

Burns

- Test the temperature of formula and bath water.
- Place pots on back burner and turn handle away from front of stove.
- Supervise the use of faucets.
- Keep matches and lighters out of reach.
- Cover electrical outlets.

PRESCHOOLERS AND SCHOOL-AGE CHILDREN

Drowning

- Be sure child has learned to swim and knows rules of water safety.
- Place locked fences around home and neighborhood pools.
- Provide supervision near pools or water.
- Teach to never swim alone and to wear a life jacket in boats.

Motor vehicle injury

- Use booster seats for children who are less than 4 feet 9 inches tall and weigh less than 40 lb (usually 4 to 8 years old). The child should be able to sit with his back against the car seat, and his legs should dangle over the seat.
- If car has a passenger air bag, place children under 12 years in the back seat.
- Use seat belts properly after booster seats are no longer necessary.
- Use protective equipment when participating in sports, riding a bike, or riding as a passenger on a bike.
- Supervise and teach safe use of equipment.
- Teach the child to play in safe areas and never to run after a ball or toy that goes into a road.
- Teach the child safety rules of the road.

Sex eduction: Begin sex education for school-age child.

Firearms

- Keep firearms unloaded, locked up, and out of reach.
- Teach to never touch a gun or stay at a friend's house where a gun is accessible.
- Store bullets in a different location from guns.

Play injury

- Teach to not run with candy or objects in mouth.
- Remove doors from refrigerators or other potentially confining structures.
- Ensure that bikes are the appropriate size for child.
- Teach playground safety.
- Teach to play in safe areas, and avoid heavy machinery, railroad tracks, excavation areas, quarries, trunks, and vacant buildings.
- Teach to avoid strangers and keep parents informed of strangers.

Burns

- Reduce setting on water heater to no higher than 49° C (120° F).
- Teach dangers of playing with matches, fireworks, and firearms.
- Teach school-age child how to properly use microwave and other cooking instruments.

Poison

- Teach child about the hazards of alcohol, cigarettes, and prescription, non-prescription, and illegal substances.
- Keep potentially dangerous substances out of reach.
- Teach parents to have the nationwide poison control number near every phone in the home and programmed in each cell phone (1-800-222-1222).

ADOLESCENTS

Motor vehicle and injury
- Ensure the teen has completed a driver's education course.
- Set rules on the number of people allowed to ride in cars, seat belt use, and to call for a ride home if a driver is impaired.
- Educate on the hazards of driving while distracted (eating or drinking, making phone calls or texting).
- Reinforce teaching on proper use of protective equipment when participating in sports.
- Teach about the hazards of firearms and safety precautions with firearms.
- Teach water safety.
- Teach to check water depth before diving.
- Be alert to indications of depression, anxiety or other behavioral changes.
- Educate on the hazards of smoking, alcohol, legal and illegal substances, and unprotected sex.
- Discuss dangers of social networking and the Internet.

Burns
- Teach to use sunblock and protective clothing.
- Teach the dangers of sunbathing and tanning beds.

YOUNG AND MIDDLE-AGE ADULTS

Motor vehicle crashes are a leading cause of death and injury to adults. Occupational injuries contribute to the injury and death rate of adults. High consumption of alcohol and suicide are also major concerns for adults.

CLIENT EDUCATION
- Remind clients to drive defensively and to not drive after drinking alcohol.
- Reinforce teaching about the long-term effects related to high alcohol consumption.
- Ensure home safety with smoke and carbon monoxide detectors, fire alarms, well-lit and uncluttered staircases.
- Be attuned to behaviors that suggest the presence of depression or thoughts of suicide. Referring clients as appropriate and encourage counseling.
- Teach diving and water safety.
- Encourage clients to become proactive about safety in the workplace and in the home.
- Discuss dangers of social networking and the Internet.
- Ensure that clients understand the hazards of excessive sun exposure and the need to protect the skin with the use of sun-blocking agents and protective clothing.

OLDER ADULTS

- The rate at which age-related changes occur varies greatly among older adults. Ⓒ
- Many older adults are able to maintain a lifestyle that promotes independence and the ability to protect themselves from safety hazards.
- Prevention is important because elderly clients can have longer recovery times from injuries and are at an increased risk for complications from injuries.
- A decrease in tactile sensitivity can place the client at risk for burns and other types of tissue injury.
- When the client demonstrates factors that increases the risk for injury (regardless of age), a home hazard evaluation should be conducted by a nurse, physical therapist, and/or occupational therapist. The client is made aware of the environmental factors that can pose a risk to safety and suggested modifications to be made.

RISK FACTORS FOR FALLS IN OLDER ADULTS
- Physical, cognitive, and sensory changes
- Changes in the musculoskeletal and neurological systems
- Impaired vision and/or hearing
- Frequent trips to the bathroom at night because of nocturia and incontinence

MODIFICATIONS TO IMPROVE HOME SAFETY
- Remove items that could cause the client to trip, such as throw rugs and loose carpets.
- Place electrical cords and extension cords against a wall behind furniture.
- Monitor gait and balance, and provide aids as needed.
- Make sure that steps and sidewalks are in good repair.
- Place grab bars near the toilet and in the tub or shower, and install a stool riser.
- Use a nonskid mat in the tub or shower.
- Wear nonskid footwear.
- Place a shower chair in the shower and provide a bedside commode if needed.
- Ensure that lighting is adequate inside and outside the home.

HOME SAFETY PLAN

FIRE

Home fires continue to be a major cause of death and injury for people of all ages. Nurses should educate clients about the importance of a home safety plan.

- Keep emergency numbers near the phone for prompt use in the event of an emergency of any type.
- Ensure that the number and placement of fire extinguishers and smoke alarms are adequate and that they are operable.
- Install and maintain smoke alarms in the home on every floor and near all rooms family members sleep in
- Set a time to routinely change the batteries in the smoke alarms (in the fall when the clocks are set to standard time and spring when set at daylight saving time).
- Have a family exit and meeting plan for fires that is reviewed and practiced regularly.
- Be sure to close windows and doors if able.
- Exit a smoke-filled area by covering the mouth and nose with a damp cloth and getting down as close to the floor as possible.
- Review with clients of all ages that in the event that the clothing or skin is on fire "stop, drop, and roll" to extinguish the fire.

SAFE USE OF OXYGEN IN THE HOME

If oxygen is used in the home, oxygen safety measures should be reviewed. Oxygen can cause materials to combust more easily and burn more rapidly, so the client and family must be provided with information on use of the oxygen delivery equipment and the dangers of combustion.

- Use and store oxygen equipment according to the manufacturer's recommendations.
- Place a "No Smoking" sign in a conspicuous place near the front door of the home. A sign can also be placed on the door to the client's bedroom.
- Inform the client and family of the danger of smoking in the presence of oxygen. Family members and visitors who smoke should do so outside the home.
- Ensure that electrical equipment is in good repair and well grounded.
- Replace bedding that generates static electricity (wool, nylon, synthetics) with items made from cotton.
- Keep flammable materials, such as heating oil and nail polish remover, away from the client when oxygen is in use.
- Follow general measures for fire safety in the home, such as having a fire extinguisher readily available and an established exit route should a fire occur.

ADDITIONAL RISKS IN THE HOME AND COMMUNITY

Additional risks in the home and community include passive smoking, carbon monoxide poisoning, and food poisoning. Bioterrorism has also become a concern, making disaster plans a mandatory part of community safety. Nurses should teach clients about the dangers of these additional risks.

Passive smoking

Passive smoking (secondhand smoke) is the unintentional inhalation of tobacco smoke.

- Exposure to nicotine and other toxins places people at risk for numerous diseases, including cancer, heart disease, and lung infections.
- Low birth weight, prematurity, stillbirths, and sudden infant death syndrome (SIDS) have been associated with maternal smoking.
- Passive smoking is associated with childhood development of bronchitis, pneumonia, and middle ear infections.
- For children who have asthma, exposure to passive smoke can result in an increase in the frequency and the severity of asthma attacks.

CLIENT EDUCATION
Nurses should inform clients who smoke and their families about the following.

- Hazards of smoking
- Resources to stop smoking (smoking-cessation programs, medication support, self-help groups)
- Effect that visiting individuals who smoke or riding in the automobile of a smoker has on a nonsmoker

Carbon monoxide

- Carbon monoxide is a very dangerous gas because it binds with hemoglobin and ultimately reduces the oxygen supplied to tissues in the body.
- Carbon monoxide cannot be seen, smelled, or tasted.
- Indications of carbon monoxide poisoning include nausea, vomiting, headache, weakness, and unconsciousness.
- Death can occur with prolonged exposure.
- Measures to prevent carbon monoxide poisoning include ensuring proper ventilation when using fuel-burning devices (lawn mowers, wood-burning and gas fireplaces, charcoal grills).
- Gas-burning furnaces, water heaters, and appliances should be inspected annually.
- Flues and chimneys should be unobstructed.
- Carbon monoxide detectors should be installed in homes and inspected regularly.
- Set a specific time to routinely change the batteries in carbon monoxide alarms.

Food poisoning

- Food poisoning is a major cause of illness in the U.S.
- Most food poisoning is caused by some bacteria, such as *Escherichia coli*, *Listeria monocytogenes*, and *salmonella*.
- Healthy individuals usually recover from the illness in a few days.
- Very young, very old, pregnant, and immunocompromised individuals are at risk for complications.
- Clients who are especially at risk are instructed to follow a low-microbial diet.
- Most food poisoning occurs because of unsanitary food practice.
- Proper hand hygiene; ensuring that eggs, meat and fish are cooked to the correct temperature; handling raw and cooked food separately to avoid cross-contamination; not using the same container, cutting board, or utensils for raw and cooked foods; refrigerating perishable items; washing raw fruits and vegetables before peeling, cutting, or eating; and not consuming unpasteurized dairy products or untreated water are measures that can prevent food poisoning.

Bioterrorism

- Bioterrorism is the dissemination of harmful toxins, bacteria, viruses, or pathogens for the purpose of causing illness or death.
- Anthrax, variola major (smallpox), *Clostridium botulinum*, *Yersinia pestis* (plague), and ricin toxin are examples of agents used by terrorists.
- Nurses and other health professionals must be prepared to respond to an attack by being proficient in early detection, recognizing the causative agent, identifying the affected community, and providing early treatment to affected people. For more information, go to the website of the Association of Professionals in Infection Control and Epidemiology (www.apic.org).

Ergonomic principles

Ergonomics are the factors or qualities in an object's design and/or use that contribute to comfort, safety, efficiency, and ease of use. **Qs**

- Body mechanics is the proper use of muscles to maintain balance, posture, and body alignment when performing a physical task. Nurses use body mechanics when providing care to clients by lifting, bending, and carrying out the activities of daily living.
- The risk of injury to the client and the nurse is reduced with the use of good body mechanics. Whenever possible, mechanical lift devices should be used to lift and transfer clients. Many health care agencies have "no manual lift" and "no solo lift" policies.

GUIDELINES TO PREVENT INJURY

- Know your agency's policies regarding lifting.
- Plan ahead for activities that require lifting, transfer, or ambulation of a client, and ask other staff members to be ready to assist at the time planned.
- Be aware that the safest way to lift a client can be with the use of assistive equipment.
- Rest between heavy lifting activities to decrease muscle fatigue.
- Maintain good posture and exercise regularly to increase the strength of arm, leg, back, and abdominal muscles so these activities require less energy.
- Use smooth movements when lifting and moving clients to prevent injury through sudden or jerky muscle movements.
- When standing for long periods of time, flex the hip and knee through use of a foot rest. When sitting for long periods of time, keep the knees slightly higher than the hips.
- Avoid repetitive movements of the hands, wrists, and shoulders. Take a break every 15 to 20 min to flex and stretch joints and muscles.
- Maintain good posture (head and neck in straight line with pelvis) to avoid neck flexion and hunched shoulders, which can cause impingement of nerves in the neck.
- Avoid twisting the spine or bending at the waist (flexion) to minimize the risk for injury.

Center of gravity

- The center of gravity is the center of a mass.
- Weight is a quantity of matter acted on by the force of gravity.
- To lift an object, the nurse must overcome the weight of the object and know the center of gravity of the object.
- When the human body is in the upright position, the center of gravity is the pelvis.
- When an individual moves, the center of gravity shifts.
- The closer the line of gravity is to the center of the base of support, the more stable the individual is.
- To lower the center of gravity, bend the hips and knees.

Lifting

- Use the major muscle groups to prevent back strain, and tighten the abdominal muscles to increase support to the back muscles.
- Distribute the weight between the large muscles of the arms and legs to decrease the strain on any one muscle group and avoid strain on smaller muscles.
- When lifting an object from the floor, flex the hips, knees, and back. Get the object to thigh level keeping the knees bent and straightening the back. Stand up while holding the object as close as possible to the body, bringing the load to the center of gravity to increase stability and decrease back strain.
- Use assistive devices whenever possible, and seek assistance whenever it is needed.

Pushing or pulling a load

- Widen the base of support.
- When opportunity allows, pull objects toward the center of gravity rather than pushing away.
- If pushing, move the front foot forward. If pulling, move the rear leg back to promote stability.
- Face the direction of movement when moving a client.
- Use own body as a counterweight when pushing or pulling, which makes the movement easier.
- Sliding, rolling, and pushing require less energy than lifting and have less risk for injury.
- Avoid twisting the thoracic spine and bending the back while the hips and knees are straight.

Transfers and use of assistive devices

- Assess the client's ability to help with transfers (balance, muscle strength, endurance).
- Determine the need for additional personnel or assistive devices (transfer belt, hydraulic lift, sliding board).
- Assess and monitor the client's use of mobility aids (canes, walkers, crutches).
- Include assistance or mobility aids needed for safe transfers and ambulation in plan of care.

Use of computers for electronic medical records

- Complete training to safely use computer and support equipment.
- Use adequate lighting.
- If adjustable, position laptop to appropriate height to be able to sit or stand while accessing or inputting data.

Application Exercises

1. A home health nurse is assessing the safety of a client's home. The nurse should identify which of the following factors as increasing the client's risk for falls? (Select all that apply.)

   A. History of a previous fall

   B. Reduced vision

   C. Impaired memory

   D. Takes rosuvastatin

   E. Uses a night light

   F. Kyphosis

2. A nurse on an acute care unit is caring for a client following a total hip arthroplasty. The client is confused, is moving his leg into positions that could dislocate the new hip joint, and he repeatedly attempts to get out of bed. After determining that restraint application is indicated, which of the following actions should the nurse take? (Select all that apply.)

   A. Secure the restraint to the frame of the bed.

   B. Get an prescription for restraints from the provider.

   C. Have a family member sign the consent for restraints.

   D. Use a square knot to secure the restraints to the bed.

   E. Ensure that only one finger can be inserted between the restraint and the client.

3. A nurse is observing a newly licensed nurse and an assistive personnel (AP) pull a client up in bed using a drawsheet. Which of the following actions by the newly licensed nurse indicates an understanding of this technique?

   A. The nurse stands with his feet together.

   B. The nurse uses his body weight to counter the client's weight.

   C. The nurse's feet are facing inward, toward the center of the bed.

   D. The nurse uses the muscles in his back to lift the client off the bed using the drawsheet.

4. A nurse is caring for a client who has diabetes mellitus and had a morning blood glucose level of 285 mg/dL. An assistive personnel (AP) reports that a client's finger-stick blood glucose reading 30 min before lunch is 58 mg/dL. Which of the following actions should the nurse take?

   A. Recheck the client's blood glucose.

   B. Complete a facility incident report.

   C. Inform the AP to give the client 120 mL of orange juice.

   D. Administer insulin as prescribed.

5. A nurse is reviewing the hospital's fire safety policies and procedures with newly hired assistive personnel. The nurse is describing what to do when there is a fire in a client's trash can. Which of the following information should the nurse include? (Select all that apply.)

   A. The first step is to pull the alarm.

   B. Use a Class C fire extinguisher to put out the fire.

   C. Instruct ambulatory clients to evacuate to a safe place.

   D. Pull the pin on the fire extinguisher prior to use.

   E. Close all doors.

PRACTICE Active Learning Scenario

A nurse manager is preparing to discuss electrical safety with the nurses on her unit. List the information that should be included in the discussion for each of the following aspects of safety. Use the ATI Active Learning Template: Basic Concept to complete this item.

UNDERLYING PRINCIPLES
- Identify the frequency in which the nurse should check equipment.
- List four measures to prevent electrical shock.

Application Exercises Key

1. A. **CORRECT:** A client who has had a previous fall is at an increased risk for another fall.

   B. **CORRECT:** Reduced vision increases the client's risk for tripping over equipment and furniture.

   C. **CORRECT:** A client who has impaired memory is at an increased risk for falls due to not asking for help with ambulation or ADLs.

   D. This medication does not place the client at risk for falls.

   E. The use of night lights and adequate lighting decreases the risk for falls.

   F. **CORRECT:** Kyphosis, which is a type of curvature of the spine, alters the client's posture and center of balance and can place the client at risk for falls.

   Ⓝ *NCLEX® Connection: Safety and Infection Control, Home Safety*

2. A. **CORRECT:** The nurse should secure the restraint to an immovable part of the bed such as the bed frame.

   B. **CORRECT:** The nurse must obtain a prescription from the provider as soon as possible, typically within 1 hr.

   C. **CORRECT:** The client's advocate or relative is legally required to be notified for the use of a restraint.

   D. A quick-release knot must be used to secure the restraint.

   E. The distance between the restraint and the client should be two finger widths.

   Ⓝ *NCLEX® Connection: Safety and Infection Control, Use of Restraints/Safety Devices*

3. A. When the nurse pulls a client up in bed, he should spread his legs apart to create a wide base of support.

   B. **CORRECT:** The nurse should use his body weight to counter the client's weight to make pulling easier.

   C. The nurse's feet should point at the head of the bed instead of the center of the bed.

   D. The nurse should use the larger muscles of the arm to lift the client.

   Ⓝ *NCLEX® Connection: Management of Care, Assignment, Delegation and Supervision*

4. A. **CORRECT:** Because the blood glucose was 285 mg/dL a few hours ago, it is unlikely that the blood glucose is 58 mg/dL at this time. The nurse should recalibrate the glucometer and recheck the client's blood glucose.

   B. It is not necessary for the nurse to complete an incident report for a change in the client's blood glucose level.

   C. Because the blood glucose was high a few hours ago, it is unlikely that the blood glucose is low enough to warrant giving the client orange juice. The nurse should assess the client prior to administering a simple carbohydrate.

   D. The nurse should avoid administering insulin to a client who has a blood glucose level of 58 mg/dL.

   Ⓝ *NCLEX® Connection: Safety and Infection Control, Safe Use of Equipment*

5. A. When a fire occurs in a client's room, the first step for the employee to take is to remove or evacuate the client from the room. The employee should know the RACE sequence: rescue the client, pull the alarm, confine the fire, and then extinguish the fire.

   B. Class A fire extinguishers are used for paper, wood, and cloth.

   C. **CORRECT:** Ambulatory clients can walk by themselves to a safe place.

   D. **CORRECT:** The fire extinguisher PASS sequence is pull the pin, aim at the base of the fire, squeeze the lever, and sweep the fire extinguisher from side to side.

   E. **CORRECT:** The employee should close all doors to contain the fire.

   Ⓝ *NCLEX® Connection: Safety and Infection Control, Accident/Error/Injury Prevention*

PRACTICE Answer

Using ATI Active Learning Template: Basic Concept

UNDERLYING PRINCIPLES
- The nurse should check all equipment at the beginning and end of each shift.
- Measures to prevent electrical shock
  - Ensure that all electrical equipment has a three-way plug and grounded outlet.
  - Ensure that outlet covers are used in areas such as pediatric and mental health units.
  - When unplugging equipment, grasp the plug, not the cord.
  - Disconnect all equipment prior to cleaning.
  - Ensure that outlets are not overcrowded.
  - Use extension cords only when absolute necessary. If used in an open area, tape the cords to the floor.

Ⓝ *NCLEX® Connection: Safety and Infection Control, Accident/Error/Injury Prevention*

When reviewing the following chapter, keep in mind the relevant topics and tasks of the NCLEX outline, in particular:

Client Needs: Safety and Infection Control

EMERGENCY RESPONSE PLAN: Use clinical decision-making/critical thinking for emergency response plan.

REPORTING OF INCIDENT/EVENT/IRREGULAR OCCURRENCE/VARIANCE: Evaluate response to error/event/occurrence.

SECURITY PLAN: Apply principles of triage and evacuation procedures/protocols.

Facility Protocols

Facility protocols refer to the plans and procedures in place to address specific issues that health care institutions face.

Nurses must understand their role in relation to development and implementation of facility protocols, including reporting incidents, disaster planning, emergency response, and security plans.

Reporting incidents

Incident reports are records of unexpected or unusual incidents that affected a client, employee, volunteer, or visitor in a health care facility.

- Facilities can also refer to incident reports as unusual occurrence or quality variance reports.
- In most states, as long as proper safeguards are employed, incident reports cannot be subpoenaed by clients or used as evidence in lawsuits.

Examples when an incident report should be filed
- Medication errors
- Procedure/treatment errors
- Equipment-related injuries/errors
- Needlestick injuries
- Client falls/injuries
- Visitor/volunteer injuries
- Threat made to client or staff
- Loss of property (dentures, jewelry, personal wheelchair)

Nurses must ensure the safety of clients' valuables. If a client is admitted to the facility and does not have a family member present, secure the client's valuables in accordance with facility policy. If an individual requests the client's valuables, the client must identify the person and give that person permission to be in possession of the valuables.

5.1 Example incident report

Incident Report
(This form should not be placed in the medical record or copied)

Date of incident: ____ Time: ____
Date form completed: ____
Name and title of person completing form: ____
Providers: 1. ____
2. ____

Location (select one)

Floor/unit: ____ Room #: ____

Administrative office	Emergency department	Nurses station	Other:
Ambulatory	Extended care facility	Obstetrics	
Birthing suite	Home	Operating room	
Blood bank	ICU	Parking areas	
Cafeteria	Labor & delivery	Pathology	
Cardiac cath	Laboratory	Pharmacy	
Central supply	Lobby	Public restroom	
Client's restroom	Medical records	Radiology	
Client's room	Medication room	Recovery room	
Dialysis	Mental health	Rehab/therapy	
EEG	Nuclear medicine	Same day surgery	
Elevator	Nursery	Stairs	

Person affected by incident (select one)

Employee	Visitor	List the below information if person is not a client
Home patient	Volunteer	Last name:
In-patient	Not applicable	First name:
Out-patient	Other:	Sex: (M/F) Age: DOB:
Provider		

Staff most closely involved in event (select one)

Intern	Security	EMS
Practical nurse	Student nurse	Physician assistant
Medical student	Surgical assistant	Certified registered nurse anesthetist
Patient care assistant	Technician	Certified registered nurse practitioner
Pharmacist	Therapist	Not applicable
Physician	Volunteer	Other:
Registered nurse	Administrative	
Resident physician	Environmental	

Incident report **1**

Site of injury (select one)

Abdomen	Ear(s)	Head	Neck
Ankle(s)	Elbow(s)	Hip(s)	Nose
Arm(s)	Eye(s)	Internal injury	Shoulder(s)
Back	Face	Knee(s)	Wrist(s)
Buttocks	Foot(feet)	Leg(s)	Not applicable
Chest	Hand(s)	Mouth	Other:

Description of incident (select one)

Abrasion	Death	Laceration	Sensory impairment
Abscess	Decubitus	Loss of property	Skin puncture
Amputation	Dislocation	Miscarriage	Skin tear
Birth injury	Edema	Necrosis	Spinal damage
Brain damage	Foreign body	Obstruction	Sprain
Burn - chemical	Fracture	Pain	Strain
Burn - electrical	Hematoma	Paralysis	Suicide
Burn - other	Hemorrhage	Perforation	Wound disruption
Circulatory impairment	Hives	Permanent disfigurement	
Coma	Hyperthermia	Poisoning	Not applicable
Concussion	Hypothermia	Rape	Other:
Contracture	Infection	Rash	
Contusion	Inflammation	Redness	
Damage to property	Injury to teeth	Self-inflicted injury	

Condition of the client prior to incident (select one)

Agitated	Dizzy	Uncooperative
Alert	Faint	Weak
Confused	Medicated	Not applicable
Disoriented	Unconscious	Other

Seen/treated by (select one)

Attending provider	On-call provider
Emergency department	Not applicable
Nurse (provider notified - no prescription received)	Other:

Treatment after incident (select one)

Received	Refused	Unknown	Not applicable

Incident report **2**

5.1 Example incident report (continued)

Quality Information

Transcription error involved? ☐ Yes ☐ No

☐ Procedure ☐ Diagnostic test ☐ Treatment related

Select all that apply

☐ Adverse outcome	☐ Foreign object left in patient	☐ Return to OR during same admission
☐ Application/removal of cast/spirit	☐ Hemorrhage	☐ Surgical checklist not completed
	☐ Inappropriate operation	☐ Transfer/moving of client
☐ Break in sterile technique	☐ Inappropriate time/sequence	☐ Wrong client
☐ Client tolerance	☐ Incorrect utensil count	☐ Wrong procedure
☐ Client refusal	☐ Lost/mishandled specimen	☐ Wrong site
☐ Consent - improper	☐ Monitoring	☐ Wrong test
☐ Consent - lack of	☐ Not prescribed	☐ Wrong treatment
☐ Delay in reporting results	☐ Omitted	☐ Unknown
☐ Delay in treatment	☐ Perforation	☐ Other:
☐ Error in reporting result	☐ Positioning	
☐ Medication	☐ Blood	

Select all that apply

☐ Break in sterile technique	☐ Incomplete additives	☐ Wrong dose
☐ Client refusal	☐ Incompatable blood	☐ Wrong flow rate
☐ Consent - improper	☐ Incorrect narcotic count	☐ Wrong medication (see below)
☐ Consent - lack of	☐ Infiltration requiring treatment	☐ Wrong route
☐ Contaminated	☐ IV conscious sedation with reversal agent given	☐ Wrong solution
☐ Contraindicated		☐ Wrong time
☐ Cross-match/typing error	☐ Medication given before culture	☐ Other:
☐ Delay in administration	☐ Mislabeled	
☐ Discontinued by client	☐ Out of date	
☐ Drug interaction	☐ Omission	
☐ Duplicated	☐ Reaction - blood	
☐ Food interaction	☐ Reaction - correct medication	Medication:
☐ Given after discontinued	☐ Reaction - incorrect medication	Name:
☐ Given without prescription	☐ Repeated attempts to start IV	Dosage:
☐ Inappropriate anesthetic	☐ Tubing not changed	Given:
☐ Inappropriate site	☐ Wrong client	Route:

Incident report **3**

Security

☐ Assault	☐ Breach of confidentiality	☐ Property loss	☐ Weapon
☐ Altercation	☐ Gun	☐ Property damage	
☐ Other:			

Miscellaneous Component (select all that apply)

☐ Blood borne exposure	☐ Provdier complaint	☐ Unknown
☐ Client/visitor/family complain	☐ Readmission in 72 hours	☐ Other:
☐ Client refused treatment	☐ Staff complaint	
☐ Elopement	☐ Unauthorized alcohol	
☐ Fire	☐ Unauthorized drugs	
☐ Left AMA	☐ Unplanned transfer to critical care	
☐ Needle stick		

Detailed description of the incident:

Incident report **5**

Fall section

Surface condition (select one if applicable) ☐ Wet ☐ Unknown ☐ Dry ☐ Other:

Circumstances related to fall (select all that apply)

☐ Ambulating - with permission	☐ From chair	☐ Slipped
	☐ From toilet	☐ Tripped
☐ Ambulating - without permission	☐ From wheelchair	☐ Unable to follow instructions
	☐ Improper footwear	☐ Visitor assisted client in ambulation without staff assistance
☐ Dizzy	☐ In shower	
☐ During assistance by staff	☐ In tub	☐ Unknown
☐ Equipment	☐ Incontinent	☐ Other:
☐ Fainted	☐ Lost balance	
☐ Found on floor	☐ Off stretcher	
☐ From bed	☐ Off table	

Client status prior to fall (complete all)

Call light on: / Risk for fall assessed before incident?
☐ Yes ☐ No ☐ N/A ☐ Yes ☐ No ☐ N/A

Restraints: / Medication?
☐ Yes ☐ No ☐ N/A ☐ Yes ☐ No
☐ Refused ☐ Removed Name:

Side rails: / Dosage:
☐ Up ☐ Down ☐ N/A Was restraint policy followed?
☐ Refused ☐ Yes ☐ No ☐ N/A

Bed position: / Was client on fall precautions?
☐ Up ☐ Down ☐ N/A ☐ Yes ☐ No ☐ N/A

Environmental component (select one if applicable) — Equipment:

☐ Disconnected	☐ No preventative maintenance	☐ Unknown
☐ Dislodged	☐ Not available	☐ Other:
☐ Equipment failure	☐ Tampered with	
☐ Equipment malfunction	☐ User error	

Device type: Model #: Serial #:

Hazardous materials and waste

☐ Spill/leak ☐ Exposure to hazardous material (specify): ☐ Other:

Utilities management

☐ Medical gasses	☐ Sewage problem	☐ Other:
☐ Medical vacuum	☐ Telephone problem	
☐ Power failure	☐ Water problem	

Incident report **4**

NURSING ROLE IN REPORTING INCIDENTS

In the event of an incident that involves a client, employee, volunteer, or visitor, the nurse's priority is to assess the individual for injuries and institute any immediate care measures necessary to decrease further injury. If the incident was client-related, notify the provider and implement additional tests or treatment as prescribed. Qs

INCIDENT REPORTS

- Should be completed by the person who identifies that an unexpected event has occurred. (This might not be the individual most directly involved in the incident.)
- Should be completed as soon as possible and within 24 hr of the incident.
- Considered confidential and are not shared with the client. (Nor is it acknowledged to the client that one was completed.)
- Not placed nor mentioned in the client's health care record. However, a description of the incident should be documented factually in the client's record.
- Include an objective description of the incident and actions taken to safeguard the client, as well as assessment and treatment of any injuries sustained.
- Forwarded to the risk management department or officer (varies by facility), possibly after being reviewed by the nurse manager.
- Provide data for performance improvement studies regarding the incidence of client injuries and care-related errors. Qoi

When completing an incident report, include:
- Client's name and hospital number (or visitor's name and address if visitor injury), along with the date, time, and location of the incident
- Factual description of the incident and injuries incurred, avoiding assumptions as to the incident's cause
- Names of witnesses to the incident and client or witness comments regarding the incident
- Corrective actions that were taken, including notification of the provider and referrals
- Name and dose of any medication or identification number of any equipment involved in the incident

Disaster planning and emergency response

A **disaster** is an event that can cause serious damage, destruction, injuries, and death. In many situations, a hospital can manage the event with the support of local resources.

A **mass casualty incident (MCI)** is a catastrophic event that overwhelms local resources. Multiple resources (federal and state) are necessary to handle the crisis.

Emergency operating plan

Each facility must have an emergency operating plan (EOP). An essential component of the plan is the provision of training of all personnel regarding each component of the EOP. Nurses should understand their responsibilities in the EOP.
- Facilities accredited by the Joint Commission must have an EOP and are mandated to test the plan at least twice a year. Qs
- The EOP should interface with local, state, and federal resources.

Internal and external emergencies

Disasters that health care facilities face include internal and external emergencies.

Internal emergencies occur within a facility and include loss of electric power or potable (drinkable) water, and severe damage or casualties related to fire, weather (tornado, hurricane), explosion, or terrorist act. Readiness includes safety and hazardous materials protocols, and infection control policies and practices.

External emergencies affect a facility indirectly and include weather (tornado, hurricane), volcanic eruptions, earthquakes, pandemic flu, chemical plant explosions, industrial accidents, building collapses, major transportation accidents, and terrorist acts (including biological and chemical warfare). Readiness includes a plan for participation in community-wide emergencies and disasters.

Disaster response agencies

Different agencies, governmental and nongovernmental, are responsible for different levels of disaster response. Agencies that have a role in disaster response include the Federal Emergency Management Agency (FEMA), CDC, U.S. Department of Homeland Security (DHS), American Red Cross, Office of Emergency Management (OEM), and the public health system.

To receive assistance with an MCI, a state must request assistance. Federal programs include the National Incident Management System, National Domestic Preparedness Organization, and Strategic National Stockpile.

Emergency designations

Health care facilities have color code designations for emergencies. These vary between institutions, but some examples are:
- Code Red: fire
- Code Pink: newborn/infant/child abduction
- Code Orange: chemical spill
- Code Blue: medical emergency
- Code Gray: tornado
- Code Black: bomb threat

In addition, some hospitals use plain language descriptions for significant alerts, such as violent situations or evacuations (example "Facility Alert: active shooter, main lobby.")

Nurses should be familiar with procedures and policies that outline proper measures to take when one of these emergencies are called.

NURSING ROLE IN DISASTER PLANNING AND EMERGENCY RESPONSE

EMERGENCY RESPONSE PLANS

- Health care institutions use a planning committee to develop emergency preparedness plans. The committee reviews information regarding the potential for various types of natural and man-made emergencies based on the characteristics of the community. The committee should also determine what resources are necessary to meet potential emergencies and include this information in the plan.
- The Hospital Incident Command System (HICS) for disaster management offers a clear structure for disaster management at the facility level. Q̲EBP
- Nurses and other members of the health care team should be involved in the development of an EOP for such emergencies. Criteria under which the EOP are activated should be clear. Roles for each employee should be outlined and administrative control determined. A designated area for the area command center should be established, as well as a person to serve as the incident control manager/commander.
- Other key roles in the EOP include a provider to manage client numbers and resources (medical command physician), an individual to prioritize treatment (triage officer) and a media liaison (community relations/public information officer).
- The nurse should create an action plan for personal family needs.

MASS CASUALTY TRIAGE Q̲Tᴄ

Principles of mass casualty triage should be followed in health care institutions involved in a mass casualty event.
- These differ from the principles of triage typically followed during provision of day-to-day services in an emergency or urgent care setting. (5.2)
- During mass casualty events, casualties are separated related to their potential for survival, and treatment is allocated accordingly. This type of triage is based on doing the greatest good for the greatest number of people.
- Nurses can find this situation very stressful because clients who are not expected to survive are cared for last.

DISCHARGE/RELOCATION OF CLIENTS

During an emergency such as a fire or a mass casualty event, nurses help make decisions regarding discharging clients or relocating them so their beds can be used for clients who have higher priority needs.

Nurses can use the following criteria when identifying which clients are stable enough to discharge.
- First, discharge or relocate ambulatory clients requiring minimal care.
- Next, make arrangement for continuation of care for clients who require some assistance, which could be provided in the home or tertiary care facility.
- Do not discharge or relocate clients who are unstable or require continuing nursing care and assessment unless they are in imminent danger.

TYPES OF EMERGENCIES

Fire

If a nurse discovers a fire that threatens the safety of a client, the nurse should use the RACE (Rescue, Alarm, Contain, Extinguish) mnemonic to guide the order of actions.

R: Rescue
Rescue the client and other individuals from the area.

A: Alarm
- Pull the fire alarm, which will activate the EMS response system.
- Systems that could increase fire spread are automatically shut down with activation of the alarm.

C: Confine
- Once the room or area is clear, close the door leading to the area where the fire is located as well as the fire doors in order to contain the fire.
- Keep fire doors closed as much as possible when moving from area to area within the facility to avoid the spread of smoke and fire.

E: Extinguish
- Attempt to extinguish small fires by using a single fire extinguisher, smothering it with a blanket, or dousing it with water (except with an electrical or grease fire).
- Complete evacuation of the area should occur if the fire cannot be extinguished.
- Attempts at extinguishing the fire should only be made when the employee has been properly trained in the safe and proper use of a fire extinguisher and when only one extinguisher is needed.

Severe thunderstorm/tornado

- Draw shades, and close drapes to protect against shattering glass.
- Lower all beds to the lowest position, and move beds away from the windows.
- Place blankets over all clients who are confined to beds.
- Close all doors.
- Relocate ambulatory clients into the hallways (away from windows) or other secure location designated by the facility.
- Do not use elevators.
- Turn on the severe weather channel to monitor severe weather warnings.

Biological incidents

- Be alert to indications of a possible bioterrorism attack because early detection and management is key. Often, the manifestations are similar to other illnesses. (5.3)
- Be alert for the appearance of a disease that does not normally occur at a specific time or place, has atypical manifestations, or occurs in a specific community or people group.
- In most instances, infection from biological agents is not spread from one client to another. Management of the incident includes recognition of the occurrence, directing personnel in the proper use of personal protective equipment, and, in some situations, decontamination and isolation.
- Use appropriate isolation measures
- Transport or move client only if needed for treatment and care.
- Take measures to protect self and others.
- Recognize indications of infection/poisoning and identify appropriate treatment interventions.

Chemical incidents

- Can occur as result of an accident or due to a purposeful action such as terrorism.
- Take measures to protect self and avoid contact.
- Assess and intervene to maintain airway, breathing, and circulation. Administer first aid as needed.
- Remove the offending chemical by undressing the client and removing all identifiable particulate matter. Provide immediate and prolonged irrigations of contaminated areas. Irrigate skin with running water, except for dry chemicals, such as lye or white phosphorus. In the case of exposure to a dry chemical, brush the agent off of clothing and skin.
- Gather a specific history of the injury, if possible (name and concentration of the chemical, duration of exposure).
- Know which facilities are open to exposed clients and which are open only to unexposed clients.
- Follow the facility's emergency response plans (personal protection measures, handling and disposal of wastes, use of space and equipment, reporting).

Hazardous material incidents

- Take measures to protect self and avoid contact.
- Approach the scene with caution.
- Identify the hazardous material with available resources (emergency response guidebook, poison control centers).
- Know the location of the Safety Data Sheet (SDS) manual.
- Try to contain the material in one place prior to the arrival of the hazardous materials team.
- Decontaminate affected individuals as much as possible at or as close as possible to the scene.
  - Don gloves, gown, mask, and shoe covers to protect self from contamination.
  - Carefully and slowly remove contaminated clothing so that deposited material does not become airborne.
  - With few exceptions, water is the universal antidote. For biological hazardous materials, wash skin with copious amounts of water and antibacterial soap.
  - Place contaminated materials into large plastic bags, and seal them.

Radiological incidents

- Amount of exposure is related to duration of exposure, distance from source, and amount of shielding.
- The facility where victims are treated should activate interventions to prevent contamination of treatment areas (floors, furniture, air vents, and ducts should be covered; radiation-contaminated waste should be disposed of according to procedural guidelines).
- Wear water-resistant gowns, double-glove, and fully cover bodies with caps, booties, masks, and goggles.
- Wear radiation or dosimetry badges to monitor the amount of radiation exposure.
- Survey clients initially with a radiation meter to determine amount of contamination.
- Decontamination with soap and water and disposable towels should occur prior to the client entering the facility. Water runoff will be contaminated and should be contained.
- After decontamination, resurvey clients for residual contamination, and continue irrigation of the skin until the client is free of all contamination.

Bomb threat

- If a bomb like device is located, do not touch it. Clear the area, and isolate the device as much as possible by closing doors, for example.
- Notify the appropriate authorities and personnel (police, administrator, director of nursing).
- Cooperate with police and others: Assist to conduct search as needed, provide copies of floor plans, have master keys available, and watch for and isolate suspicious objects such as packages and boxes.
- Keep elevators available for authorities.
- Remain calm and alert and try not to alarm clients.

When a phone call is received
- Extend the conversation as long as possible.
- Listen for distinguishing background noises (music, voices, traffic, airplanes).
- Note distinguishing voice characteristics of the caller.
- Ask where and when the bomb is set to explode.
- Note whether the caller is familiar with the physical arrangement of the facility.

5.2 Categories of triage during mass casualty

Emergent (CLASS I)	Urgent (CLASS II)	Nonurgent (CLASS III)	Expectant (CLASS IV)
Highest priority is given to clients who have life-threatening injuries but also have a high possibility of survival once they are stabilized.	Second-highest priority is given to clients who have major injuries that are not yet life-threatening and usually can wait 45 to 60 min for treatment.	The next highest priority is given to clients who have minor injuries that are not life-threatening and do not need immediate attention.	The lowest priority is given to clients who are not expected to live and will be allowed to die naturally. Comfort measures can be provided, but restorative care will not.

Security plans

- All facilities should have security plans in place that include preventive, protective, and response measures designed for identified security needs.
- Security issues faced by health care facilities include admission of potentially dangerous individuals, vandalism, infant abduction, and information theft.
- The International Association for Healthcare Security & Safety (IAHSS) provides recommendations for the development of security plans.

NURSING ROLE IN SECURITY PLANS

Nurses should be prepared to take immediate action when breaches in security occur. Time is of the essence in preventing a breach in security. Qs

SECURITY MEASURES

- An identification system that identifies employees, volunteers, physicians, students, and regularly scheduled contract services staff as authorized personnel of the facility
- Electronic security systems in high-risk areas (the maternal newborn unit to prevent infant abductions, the emergency department to prevent unauthorized entrance)
  - Key code access into and out of high-risk areas
  - Wrist bands that electronically link parents and their infant
  - Alarms integrated with closed-circuit television cameras

5.3 Biological incidents and their treatment and prevention

Inhalational anthrax
MANIFESTATIONS
- Fever
- Cough
- Shortness of breath
- Muscle aches
- Mild chest pain
- Meningitis
- Shock

PREVENTION: Anthrax vaccine for high-risk; ciprofloxacin & doxycycline IV/PO

TREATMENT: Includes one or two additional antibiotics such as vancomycin, penicillin and anthrax antitoxin

Cutaneous anthrax
MANIFESTATIONS
- Starts as a lesion that can be itchy
- Develops into a vesicular lesion that later becomes necrotic with the formation of black eschar
- Fever, chills

PREVENTION: Anthrax vaccine for high-risk

TREATMENT: Ciprofloxacin, doxycycline

Botulism
MANIFESTATIONS
- Difficulty swallowing
- Double vision
- Slurred speech
- Descending progressive weakness
- Nausea, vomiting, abdominal cramps
- Difficulty breathing

PREVENTION/TREATMENT
- Airway management
- Antitoxin
- Elimination of toxin

Viral hemorrhagic fevers
Examples: Ebola, yellow fever

MANIFESTATIONS
- Sore throat
- Headache
- High temperature
- Nausea, vomiting, diarrhea
- Internal and external bleeding
- Shock

PREVENTION: vaccination available for yellow fever, Argentine hemorrhagic fever; barrier protection from infected person, isolation precautions specific to disease

TREATMENT: no cure, supportive care only; minimize invasive procedures

Plague
MANIFESTATIONS
- Forms can occur separately or in combination
- Pneumonic: fever, headache, weakness, pneumonia with shortness of breath, chest pain, cough, and bloody or watery sputum
- Bubonic: swollen, tender lymph glands, fever, headache, chills, and weakness
- Septicemic: fever, chills, prostration, abdominal pain, shock, disseminated intravascular coagulation, gangrene of nose and digits

PREVENTION: Contact precautions until decontaminated; droplet precautions till 72 hr after antibiotics

TREATMENT: Streptomycin/gentamicin or tetracycline/doxycycline

Smallpox
MANIFESTATIONS
- High fever
- Fatigue
- Severe headache
- Rash
- Chills
- Vomiting
- Delirium

PREVENTION: vaccine; can vaccinate within 3 days of exposure; contact and airborne precautions

TREATMENT: supportive care (prevent dehydration, provide skin care, medications for pain and fever); antibiotics for secondary infections

Tularemia
MANIFESTATIONS
- Sudden fever, chills, headache, diarrhea, muscle aches, joint pain, dry cough, progressive weakness
- If airborne, life-threatening pneumonia and systemic infection

PREVENTION: Vaccine under review by the FDA

TREATMENT: Streptomycin or gentamicin are drugs of choice; in mass causality, use doxycycline or ciprofloxacin

Application Exercises

1. A nurse discovers that a client was administered an antihypertensive medication in error. Identify the appropriate sequence of steps that the nurse should take using the following actions.

   A. Call the provider.

   B. Check vital signs.

   C. Notify the risk manager.

   D. Complete an incident report.

   E. Instruct the client to remain in bed until further notice.

2. A nurse manager is explaining the use of incident reports to a group of nurses in an orientation program. Which of the following information should the nurse manager include? (Select all that apply.)

   A. A description of the incident should be documented in the client's health care record.

   B. The client should sign as a witness on the incident report.

   C. Incident reports include a description of the incident and actions taken.

   D. A copy of the incident report should be placed in the client's health care record.

   E. The risk management department investigates the incident.

3. A nurse is discussing disaster planning with the board members of a hospital. Which of the following individuals should the nurse expect to request extra supplies and staffing for the facility?

   A. Incident commander

   B. Medical command physician

   C. Triage officer

   D. Media liaison

4. A community experiences an outbreak of meningitis, and hospital beds are urgently needed. Which of the following clients should the nurse recommend for discharge?

   A. A client newly admitted with angina and a history of myocardial infarction 1 year ago

   B. A client who has type 2 diabetes mellitus and was admitted for rotator cuff surgery

   C. A client admitted the day before with pneumonia and dehydration

   D. A client who has a fractured hip and is scheduled for total hip replacement the next day

5. A nurse on a sixth-floor medical-surgical unit is advised that a severe weather alert code has been activated. Which of the following actions should the nurse take? (Select all that apply.)

   A. Open window shades or drapes to provide better visibility of the external environment.

   B. Move beds of nonambulatory clients away from windows.

   C. Relocate ambulatory clients into the hallways.

   D. Use the elevators to move clients to lower levels.

   E. Turn the radio on for severe weather warnings.

PRACTICE Active Learning Scenario

A nurse serving on a disaster preparedness committee is reviewing information about smallpox. Use the ATI Active Learning Template: System Disorder to complete this item.

EXPECTED FINDINGS: List at least three manifestations.

THERAPEUTIC PROCEDURES: List at least two treatment measures.

Application Exercises Key

1. Correct order

   B. The first action the nurse should take using the nursing process is to monitor the client for hypotension by checking vital signs.

   E. Next, the nurse should instruct the client to remain in bed to prevent a fall due to the risk of hypotension.

   A. Then the nurse should notify the provider, who may prescribe a medication to treat hypotension.

   D. Next, the nurse should complete an incident report that is thorough, objective, and accurate.

   C. The last step the nurse should take is to report the incident to the risk manager.

   Ⓝ *NCLEX® Connection: Safety and Infection Control, Reporting of Incident/Event/Irregular Occurrence Variance*

2. A. **CORRECT:** The nurse should document a factual description of the event in the client's health care record.

   B. The nurse should not inform the client or individual involved that an incident report has been filed. Incident reports are for facility quality assurance.

   C. **CORRECT:** In addition to providing an accurate description of the event, the nurse also should document the actions taken following the event.

   D. The nurse should not place the incident report in the client's health care record in order to shield it from discovery in the event of a lawsuit.

   E. **CORRECT:** The nurse should expect a risk manager to investigate all incidents as part of the agency's quality assurance program.

   Ⓝ *NCLEX® Connection: Safety and Infection Control, Reporting of Incident/Event/Irregular Occurrence Variance*

3. A. The nurse should expect the incident commander to manage the incident and key leaders within the facility.

   B. **CORRECT:** The nurse should expect the medical command physician to oversee use of resources such as equipment and personnel.

   C. The nurse should expect the triage officer to prioritize the treatment of incoming clients

   D. The nurse should expect the media liaison to communicate with members of the media and press on behalf of the facility.

   Ⓝ *NCLEX® Connection: Safety and Infection Control, Emergency Response Plan*

4. A. The nurse should recognize that a client who has angina is at risk for a cardiac event. The nurse should not recommend this client for discharge because the client is unstable.

   B. **CORRECT:** The nurse should identify that this client is stable and his condition can be managed at home with surgery rescheduled. The nurse can safely recommend this client for discharge.

   C. The nurse should recognize a client who has dehydration and active infection requires ongoing nursing care. The nurse should not recommend this client for discharge because the client is unstable.

   D. The nurse should recognize that a client who has hip fracture is unstable, and at risk for further damage to her hip. The nurse should not recommend this client for discharge because the client is unstable.

   Ⓝ *NCLEX® Connection: Safety and Infection Control, Emergency Response Plan*

5. A. The nurse should close the window shades and drapes to protect clients from shattering glass.

   B. **CORRECT:** The nurse should move the beds of nonambulatory clients away from windows to protect clients from shattering glass.

   C. **CORRECT:** The nurse should relocate ambulatory clients into the hallway to protect the clients from shattering glass.

   D. The nurse should instruct others that it is unsafe to use the elevator.

   E. **CORRECT:** The nurse should use the radio to monitor the activity of the storm.

   Ⓝ *NCLEX® Connection: Safety and Infection Control, Emergency Response Plan*

PRACTICE Answer

Using ATI Active Learning Template: System Disorder

EXPECTED FINDINGS	THERAPEUTIC PROCEDURES
• High fever	• Prevent dehydration.
• Fatigue	• Provide skin care.
• Severe headache	• Administer medications for pain and fever.
• Rash	• Provide vaccination if within 3 days of exposure.
• Chills	• Implement contact and airborne precautions.
• Vomiting	• Administer antibiotics for secondary infections.
• Delirium	

Ⓝ *NCLEX® Connection: Safety and Infection Control, Emergency Response Plan*

References

Berman, A., Snyder, S., & Frandsen, G. (2016). *Kozier & Erb's fundamentals of nursing: Concepts, process, and practice* (10th ed.). Upper Saddle River, NJ: Prentice-Hall.

Cherry, B., & Jacob, S. R. (2014). *Contemporary nursing: Issues, trends, & management* (6th ed.). St. Louis, MO: Mosby, Inc.

Eliopoulos, C. (2014). *Gerontological nursing* (8th ed.). Philadelphia: Lippincott Williams & Wilkins.

Halter, M. J. (2014). *Varcarolis' foundations of psychiatric mental health nursing: A clinical approach* (7th ed.). St. Louis, MO: Saunders.

Marquis, B. L., & Huston, C. J. (2015). *Leadership roles and management functions in nursing: Theory and application* (8th ed.). Philadelphia: Lippincott Williams & Wilkins.

Potter, P. A., Perry, A. G., Stockert, P., & Hall, A. (2013). *Fundamentals of nursing* (8th ed.). St. Louis, MO: Mosby.

Stanhope, M., & Lancaster, J. (2014). *Foundations of nursing in the community* (4th ed.). St. Louis, MO: Mosby.

Weiss, S. A., & Tappen, R. M. (2015). *Essentials of nursing leadership & management* (6th ed.). Philadelphia: F.A. Davis Company.

STUDENT NAME _____

CONCEPT_____ REVIEW MODULE CHAPTER_____

Related Content
(E.G., DELEGATION,
LEVELS OF PREVENTION,
ADVANCE DIRECTIVES)

Underlying Principles

Nursing Interventions
WHO? WHEN? WHY? HOW?

ACTIVE LEARNING TEMPLATE: Diagnostic Procedure

STUDENT NAME _____

PROCEDURE NAME _____ REVIEW MODULE CHAPTER_____

Description of Procedure

Indications

CONSIDERATIONS

Nursing Interventions (pre, intra, post)

Interpretation of Findings

Client Education

Potential Complications

Nursing Interventions

STUDENT NAME _____

DEVELOPMENTAL STAGE _____ REVIEW MODULE CHAPTER_____

EXPECTED GROWTH AND DEVELOPMENT

Physical Development	Cognitive Development	Psychosocial Development	Age-Appropriate Activities

Health Promotion

Immunizations	Health Screening	Nutrition	Injury Prevention

STUDENT NAME _____

MEDICATION _____ REVIEW MODULE CHAPTER_____

CATEGORY CLASS_____

PURPOSE OF MEDICATION

Expected Pharmacological Action

Therapeutic Use

Complications

Medication Administration

Contraindications/Precautions

Nursing Interventions

Interactions

Client Education

Evaluation of Medication Effectiveness

STUDENT NAME _____

SKILL NAME_____ REVIEW MODULE CHAPTER_____

Description of Skill

Indications

CONSIDERATIONS

Nursing Interventions (pre, intra, post)

Outcomes/Evaluation

Client Education

Potential Complications

Nursing Interventions

System Disorder

STUDENT NAME _____

DISORDER/DISEASE PROCESS _____ REVIEW MODULE CHAPTER_____

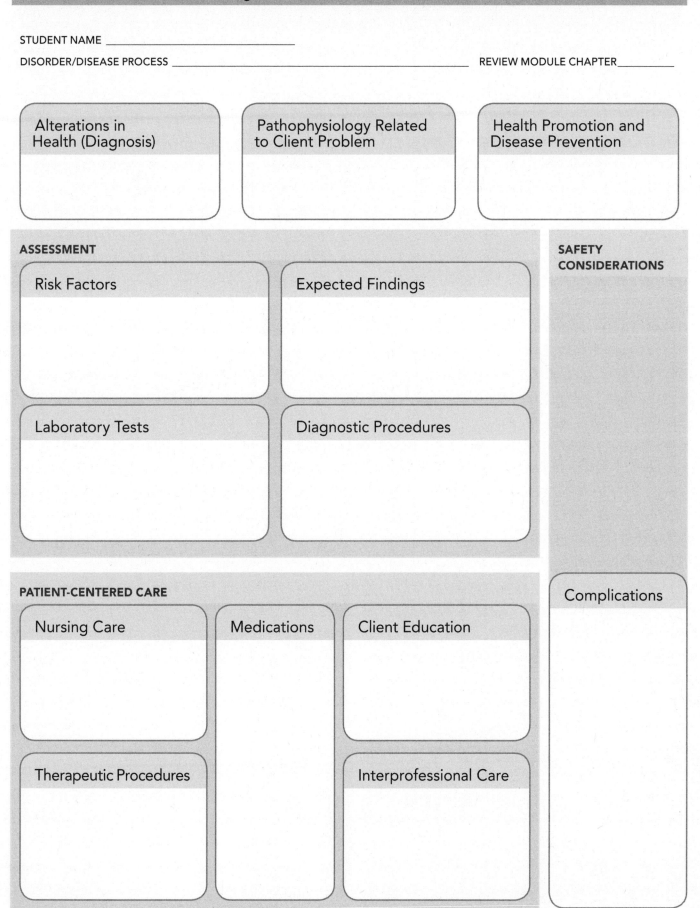

Alterations in Health (Diagnosis)

Pathophysiology Related to Client Problem

Health Promotion and Disease Prevention

ASSESSMENT

SAFETY CONSIDERATIONS

Risk Factors

Expected Findings

Laboratory Tests

Diagnostic Procedures

PATIENT-CENTERED CARE

Complications

Nursing Care

Medications

Client Education

Therapeutic Procedures

Interprofessional Care

ACTIVE LEARNING TEMPLATE: *Therapeutic Procedure*

STUDENT NAME _____

PROCEDURE NAME _____ REVIEW MODULE CHAPTER_____

Description of Procedure

Indications

CONSIDERATIONS

Nursing Interventions (pre, intra, post)

Outcomes/Evaluation

Client Education

Potential Complications

Nursing Interventions